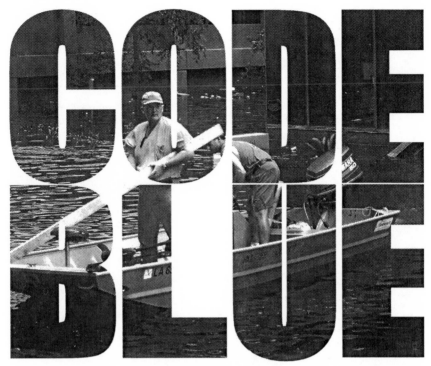

A KATRINA PHYSICIAN'S MEMOIR

Richard E. Deichmann, M.D.

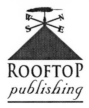

ROOFTOP
publishing

Rooftop Publishing™
1663 Liberty Drive, Suite 200
Bloomington, IN 47403
Phone: 1-800-839-8640

This book is a work of non-fiction. Unless otherwise noted, the author and the publisher make no explicit guarantees as to the accuracy of the information contained in this book and in some cases, names of people and places have been altered to protect their privacy.

First published by Rooftop Publishing 03/21/2007

ISBN: 978-1-60008-026-5 (sc)

Library of Congress Control Number: 2007924430

Printed in the United States of America
Bloomington, Indiana

This book is printed on acid-free paper.

*For those who suffered through the
post-Katrina flood at Baptist Hospital*

The official name of Baptist Hospital was Memorial Medical Center. I refer to it as Baptist Hospital, since this was its original name, and the one that most staff and patients continue to use when referring to the institution. All of the events described are as true as my admittedly fallible memory allows. Several names have been changed, but the events portrayed in the story are real.

INTRODUCTION:

The Storm Was Named Katrina

As I reluctantly adjusted to the life of a refugee in Atlanta a few weeks after the storm, I opened the newspaper one morning to find the headlines boldly announcing the "gruesome discovery" at Baptist Hospital. Forty-five bodies had been found at the facility after the eight feet of water surrounding the facility had receded. Images of the bodies in the chapel made it into newspapers and televisions around the country. About the same time, the Louisiana state attorney general announced that he would investigate charges of euthanasia occurring at the hospital.

A media feeding frenzy ensued. Radio, television, and newspaper reporters tracked me down in Atlanta to get my "reaction" to the allegations of euthanasia. The sensational media coverage of the allegations spun the story in ways very different from what I remember happening during those dark days in Baptist Hospital.

I was there.

When my wife Cecile and I left New Orleans on Tuesday, August 22, 2005, to bring our oldest daughter Beth to college for the first time, a hurricane was the furthest thing from my mind. My main concern was if I had the dorm room refrigerator secured well enough to the roof rack on the car. The inside of the SUV was stacked to the ceiling with clothes, pictures, electronics, and more clothes. We set off for an overnight stay in Atlanta with Cecile's sister Meredith, on our way to Chapel Hill, North Carolina. Our other two teenage daughters, Claire and Paige, stayed behind at the house alone. Our neighbors and their grandmother served as surrogate parents if they got into trouble. Our plan included a short stay in our family home in Highlands, North Carolina, on our way back to New Orleans after helping Beth settle into the dorm. We'd drive back home on Monday.

We pulled up to Granville Towers at UNC in Chapel Hill after dark, worn out from the two-day trip. After unloading the car into one dorm room, we had to move all the stuff into another room, after discovering black mold in the first room. The three of us had a late dinner with Carl and Mandy—Cecile's brother and sister-in-law, who lived in Durham—and then brought Beth back to the dorm. By the time we got to Carl and Mandy's house around midnight, we collapsed into bed like wet noodles.

We spent Thursday roaming the campus, listening to "Welcome to Carolina" seminars, and watching student organization presentations. A beautiful Carolina-blue sky gleaned above. Cecile and I reminisced about the years of laughter we had enjoyed in Chapel Hill. We had met at Tulane Medical School as medical students, and went to UNC School of Medicine for our residencies. We spent the first years of our marriage, almost twenty-five years ago, in this town, enjoying the food, music, and ambience. Once we finished our residencies at UNC, we moved back to New Orleans, where we both had grown up.

We helped Beth organize her room, which had boxes and boxes strewn about from the night before. Her new roommate arrived with an even greater volume of college survival essentials than Beth had brought. I wondered how they would ever fit it all in the room. We all swapped stories and got to know each other a little. Beth and her roommate joked about their college experience so far, which was only twenty-four hours old. Cecile, Beth, and I made the requisite trip to Wal-Mart to pick up extension cords, hangers, a backrest, and other basics of college life. That evening, we enjoyed another meal with Carl and Mandy, and then drove Beth back to Granville.

When I got back to Carl's house Thursday night, we all cracked open a cold beer and celebrated our first daughter starting college.

"Sorry to spoil the fun," Carl said in his typically understated manner. "But I heard there's a hurricane out there that you might want to check out."

"Where'd you hear that?" I asked.

"On the TV weather report this evening. You can check it out on the Internet if you want."

I walked over to his computer in the other room and tried to get on the Internet.

"Hey, Carl. How do I get on this thing?" I yelled out to him.

Carl walked in, and within seconds, the National Hurricane Center's Web site glowed before me.

The storm was named Katrina.

The hurricane was already a Category 4 storm, and it looked like it could be headed toward New Orleans. The National Hurricane Center's early predictions pegged it going further east, toward Florida. They also predicted additional strengthening. The storm was still hundreds of miles from the mainland. The satellite pictures showed a massive swirl of clouds about a thousand miles in diameter, with a small bull's-eye in its center. I went to bed with just a slight unease. I wasn't too concerned. Anything could happen with a storm that far away. I'd check out the reports in the morning, and call New Orleans to see what was happening there.

While sipping my coffee Friday morning, I looked over the latest bulletins from the National Hurricane Center again. Katrina was still far away, but aiming toward the central Gulf Coast. I told Cecile of the news, and she agreed that we should most likely cancel the plans for Highlands and go back home if the storm didn't change course. In twenty-four hours, we went from a happy nervousness over Beth's first days at college to a set of ominous concerns about a hurricane bearing down on New Orleans.

We met with Beth again that morning to help her with another day of starting her new life in Chapel Hill. She was also caught off guard by the news about the hurricane. We spent the day opening a bank account, registering for her first-semester courses, and getting her new computer set up. All the while, my thoughts were dominated by what was happening with the storm, and how my daughters in New Orleans were handling things.

Cecile called her mother to hear about her plans. Anne told her that she and Carroll, her husband, didn't have any intention to evacuate. They felt perfectly safe and would be glad to have Claire and Paige stay with them. Anne confirmed the buzz of nervousness that had overtaken the city. Although the storm hardly made any news in Chapel Hill, I knew that everyone in New Orleans was probably glued to the TV. The low-grade fear started to seep into our spirits too.

Before leaving Beth that afternoon, we said our good-byes, in case we couldn't see her for breakfast the next morning. Cecile and I left for Carl's house and for an update from his computer about the storm.

After seeing the latest reports from the Internet Friday evening, we knew we had to leave. Katrina was aimed at New Orleans, though its course was still predicted to veer easterly. The storm was intensifying, and was predicted to grow to a Category 5 hurricane. A voluntary evacuation had been called for, and hundreds of thousands of people were leaving with their pets and belongings. The state had instituted contra-flow on interstate highways, so that soon, all lanes of the highway would be diverted to one-way roads heading away from New Orleans.

The city had been bracing for the "Big One" ever since Hurricane Betsy had pummeled it in 1965. A sophisticated system of levees and pumps encircled the entire region. Civil authorities had thick volumes of emergency hurricane plans that they regularly updated but never needed to fully implement.

Despite the many efforts to provide sound hurricane protection to the region, some authorities pointed to nagging lapses in the system. These experts noted that the steady disappearance of the marshland could make the area more vulnerable to a storm surge, which might overtop the levees. The Army Corps of Engineers knew that the levees themselves were sinking and were below specifications. Other experts pointed out that the system of pumps might not have the capacity to quickly pump out the massive amounts of rain carried by a large system. Even heavy, non-tropical rainstorms would pelt the city and regularly flood city streets.

Political forces conspired with these natural ones to make New Orleans particularly vulnerable to a hurricane disaster. The federal government had cut funding of the levee protection system over the decades. The feds also diverted the state's National Guard to Iraq and as a result, they would be unavailable in a post-hurricane crisis. Local and state officials used the local levee boards—which were charged with maintaining the levees—as political rewards for friends. Although the Corps of Engineers had ultimate responsibility for the system, no one really knew where their responsibility ended and the local levee board's began.

Weighing all the factors with each approaching hurricane over the years, I had always felt secure in my home against hurricanes. We had never evacuated for any of them. In fact, for hurricanes Georges and Ivan, we were out of town and drove back to the city to be in our home and community in case our services were needed. By the time August 2005 had rolled around, several named storms and hurricanes had already come and gone. None had seriously threatened New Orleans, and our family had not run through our usual hurricane drill.

We toyed with the idea of leaving Chapel Hill Friday night, but knew we were too tired to try to drive all night. We decided to begin the fourteen-hour drive back home at daybreak on Saturday. If we made good time, we could be home around nightfall. Since the interstates near New Orleans were diverted to outgoing traffic only, we would have to take slower, alternate routes once we got to within about fifty miles of home.

We bid our farewells to Carl and Mandy over some wine that night. They would be asleep when we left in the morning. We told Beth of our plan to skip breakfast with her in the morning and get an early start on the trip home. Once our bags were packed and the alarm set for five, we went to bed.

After a restless night, I awoke and went straight to the computer to catch the latest news. My hopes for a miracle faded as I read the reports. Katrina was a Category 4 hurricane with sustained winds in excess of 140 miles per hour. The massive system pushed a storm surge of eighteen feet. The killer hurricane still tracked a path toward New Orleans.

I chomped down on a bagel and had an extra cup of coffee for breakfast. Cecile and I hunkered down in the SUV as the sun came up, and we made for New Orleans. Along the way, we formulated our plan. I felt a responsibility to help the community and the patients in the hospital at which I worked. I didn't want to desert the area in its time of need. As the chief of the medicine department at the hospital, I felt a particular obligation to be there. Since we both wanted to care for our daughters also, the safest course seemed for our family to evacuate to the hospital until the storm passed, and then go back home. Baptist Hospital would have power, water, food, and safety behind the heavy brick walls of its multiple buildings.

Paige, our youngest daughter, called with the news that almost everyone in our neighborhood had evacuated. The two neighbors who remained were planning on leaving soon too. More than a million people were leaving or had left southeast Louisiana. I told her of our plan to evacuate to Baptist. I asked her to start getting the things together that she wanted to bring with her, and to tell Claire to do the same. Paige demanded that all the pets had to come too.

By the time we got to Mobile, warnings of the closure of I-10 westbound near New Orleans flashed from the shoulder of the road. Shortly before the Louisiana border, we turned off the interstate and made our way to the city via Highway 90. After entering Orleans Parish (Louisiana has parishes, rather than counties), the two-lane highway crosses the Rigolets, the waterway connecting the Gulf of Mexico with Lake Pontchartrain, by a drawbridge. As we approached, a large shrimp boat was puttering through the open drawbridge to safe harbor.

Cecile and I got out of our car and joined the others looking out over the bridge to the swamps beyond. As I leaned on the concrete railing of the bridge, a light sea breeze tussled what little hair I have left. The sun inched close to the horizon, sending reflections of light off the water and shadows through the tall marsh grass. To the south, a gray, heavy, overcast sky merged indistinctly with the water and swamp below. The air dripped with a lusty tropical humidity.

Katrina was out there, taking aim directly at that very spot. No one on the Rigolets Bridge that evening could have dreamed of what she had in store.

CHAPTER 1

Sunday

Louisiana, Louisiana—They're tryin' to wash us away.

— Randy Newman from "Louisiana 1927"

As we approached the Baptist Hospital parking garage, a checkpoint with three security guards at the entrance made it clear that this was not business as usual. A line of cars seeking safety from the hurricane inched its way forward to get clearance to enter the seven-story garage. With me in the lead, our two-car caravan finally arrived at the gate. A burly hospital security guard approached me. Beads of sweat glistened on her dark skin. The cap barely contained her stiff brown hair. She took two steps to my car and, recognizing me, made the ritual request for my physician identification. I presented my credentials to her. She looked in my car. My two teenage daughters, Claire and Paige, sat in the back seat, motionless. Their eyes were still swollen from the tears of this morning's events. Claire, sporting the perfect tan she carefully nurtured throughout the summer, had not said a word since getting in the car. Paige—younger and taller than her sister—propped a bag of clothes on her runner's legs. She stayed quiet to avoid crying all over again. The guard saw the rabbit cage, the cat, two book sacks, sleeping bags, pillows, luggage, and blankets, and just shook her head. She had been peering into people's lives all morning, observing those precious things that people chose not to leave behind.

"Okay, Dr. Deichmann, you can go on in," she said.

"Officer," I said, "my wife's in the car behind me, and I was hoping you'd let her in too."

"Oooh, it be really packed inside, but I'll let her in. Maybe y'all can find a place on the second floor in the doctors' area. If you got to, just park illegally. Anywhere you find."

"Thanks."

I followed the line of cars snaking their way through the garage. My wife, Cecile, stayed right behind, ready to get our second car to higher ground.

In the past, hundreds of neighborhood residents had sought refuge for themselves and their cars at the hospital for hurricanes or even big rainstorms. The part of town that Baptist Hospital occupied was one of the lowest parts of the entire area. Sometimes heavy rainfalls would swamp the streets for hours. I'd already experienced being trapped at the hospital overnight on two occasions when the water was too high to drive a car out of the garage. Over the last two years, the flooding situation improved, after a massive drainage project had been completed in the area. No significant flooding occurred since that project's completion. Still, people knew that Katrina might be the big one. No one was taking any chances.

The sprawling complex of buildings sat where Uptown meets Broadmoor, near the corner of Napoleon and Claiborne avenues. The main hospital, the Magnolia parking garage, and the helipad occupied an entire city block. On the hospital's south side, across Magnolia Street, sat the four-story building where all surgeries and cardiac procedures were performed. An elevated, enclosed crosswalk connected this building to the hospital. Clara Street bounded the north side of the hospital. Another enclosed crosswalk over Clara Street connected the hospital to the multi-story McFarland Building. From there, an internal corridor connected the McFarland Building to the nine-story Napoleon Medical Plaza office building further north, where my office was located. A second large parking garage on the north side of the hospital was linked to the hospital by another crosswalk. Two more enclosed crosswalks spanned Jena Street at different places, to connect the garage with the Napoleon Medical Plaza building and the McFarland Building. My office was a fifteen-minute hike from the parts of the complex furthest away.

The noon weather report was giving the latest update on Hurricane Katrina as we searched for a parking spot. The National Weather Service reported that the storm—which had been a Category 5 storm hours before—was still a powerful Category 4 hurricane, with maximum winds of 140 miles per hour. The storm surge was predicted to be twenty feet. Even more ominously, the Weather Service cautioned that levees in the New Orleans area might be "overtopped." The massive system was heading directly for New Orleans.

We eventually parked illegally in two reserved spaces, just as the guard had suggested. Hundreds of others had already taken up temporary quarters and were unloading their cars. The garage was filled with people, pets, and suitcases. I grabbed the rabbit's cage, and the two girls brought in their bags. Cecile, petite yet strong, carried her belongings and the bag of food. The plan was for them to set themselves up in my office on the eighth floor of the medical office building, while I checked in at the hospital.

As chairman of the medicine department, I went to the administrative offices on the first floor, where we had practiced our crisis management exercises about three months before. Along the way, a hodgepodge of people had taken up residence in the hallways, lobbies, and common areas. Kids were laughing and tossing a Frisbee to each other. Two other grade-school kids played tag. Makeshift bedding covered out-of-the-way corners in hallways and common areas. Some adults relaxed as they puffed on their cigarettes in the non-smoking facility. Pet owners were busy walking their dogs in the hall or otherwise caring for their animals. The place had the feel of a scout campout, though it was the most unlikely campground the scouts could ever imagine.

The disaster-team members were standing around the massive conference table in the center of the room. About a dozen senior leaders mulled about, but the chief of the medical staff was absent. Susan Mulderick, a nurse administrator, was the head of the crisis team and was getting the first disaster meeting organized. Susan had been a nurse at Baptist for as long as I could remember, taking on various leadership roles along the way. Her tall, upright posture and no-nonsense manner had an authoritative, military style to it. She commanded respect and attention, and yet had a warm, disarming smile.

René Goux, the CEO, stood next to her. René had been on the job at Baptist for about a year. Before then, he had served on the hospital administrator circuit at a number of Tenet hospitals for years. With his Cajun accent and easy demeanor, he had now found his way back to his hometown, where he hoped to end his career and eventually retire.

Sean Fowler, the COO, lounged around by the food in the back of the room. Sean, aggressive and assertive, had lost his job as CEO at a nearby Tenet hospital a few months earlier when the company closed the hospital. René brought him over to Baptist and assigned him the unpleasant task of dealing with the medical staff and the daily operational problems. His husky build and short, stocky neck made him the perfect bulldog to protect the company's interests.

Dr. John Walsh, the chairman of the surgery department, was present, sporting a clean set of green scrubs. John and I had started practicing together at Baptist almost twenty years ago.

We had both graduated from Jesuit High School, Tulane College, and Tulane Medical School. We were in the same multi-specialty group when we both started practicing, but went our separate ways when the group went out of business. He loved to joke about our days at Tulane and the crazy things we got ourselves into. One of my geriatric patients once told me how she thought John was so handsome, with his curly black hair and easy, pleasant smile. He could make me laugh so hard, my facial muscles would be sore the rest of the day. John was a trusted friend and an excellent surgeon. More importantly, he was cool under fire and not prone to rash decisions.

The security director gave his report on the crowded conditions in the hospital. He reported that for every staff member, there were five accompanying family members. People from the neighborhood were still pouring into the hospital. The parking garage was full, and they decided to close it to any more vehicles. They had been putting wristbands on individuals who had legitimate access to the facility, but many people had gotten in through its porous borders without any wristbands or official accounting. After some discussion, the administrators decided to limit access to the hospital as much as possible. From this point on, the hospital would not give shelter to anyone arriving by car. Evacuees arriving on foot would be given access. The team also decided to get an accurate count of people in the hospital, and to identify everyone with special color-coded wristbands.

Next, the cook gave a summary of the food and water supplies. He was confident of at least a one-week supply of food. Of course, a lot depended on an accurate count of the number of mouths he needed to feed. Engineering reported that plenty of fuel was available for the generators, but serious flooding might knock out the switches leading to them. Other team members updated us on their areas of responsibility.

Finally, Sean reported to me on the number of physicians who had checked in to volunteer for duty. He gave me a list of the names of about twenty-five physicians who were available to help out. He then told me where they were assigned lodging, and how to contact them. He assigned a room to me in the McFarland Building and wrote down his contact information, should I need to get in touch with him. Before we disbanded, René and the cook agreed that the kitchen—which was located in the basement—would need to be moved to higher ground. The CEO's Cajun instincts knew that safeguarding the food was a key priority. We all agreed to immediately begin moving the tons of food and water to the fourth floor. A hallway and rooms there would serve as the pantry and service area for the time being. The team would assemble again that afternoon.

The meeting adjourned.

I checked the latest reports from the National Weather Service on the Internet before I left. The computer screen flickered the following warning, issued about two hours before:

URGENT - WEATHER MESSAGE

NATIONAL WEATHER SERVICE NEW ORLEANS LA

1011 A.M. CDT SUN AUG 28 2005...DEVASTATING DAMAGE EXPECTED... HURRICANE KATRINA... A MOST POWERFUL HURRICANE WITH UNPRECEDENTED STRENGTH...RIVALING THE INTENSITY OF HURRICANE CAMILLE OF 1969. MOST OF THE AREA WILL BE UNINHABITABLE FOR WEEKS...PERHAPS LONGER. AT LEAST ONE HALF OF WELL CONSTRUCTED HOMES WILL HAVE ROOF AND WALL FAILURE. ALL GABLED ROOFS WILL FAIL...LEAVING THOSE HOMES SEVERELY DAMAGED OR DESTROYED. THE MAJORITY OF INDUSTRIAL BUILDINGS WILL BECOME NON FUNCTIONAL. PARTIAL TO COMPLETE WALL AND ROOF FAILURE IS EXPECTED. ALL WOOD FRAMED LOW RISING APARTMENT BUILDINGS WILL BE DESTROYED.

CONCRETE BLOCK LOW RISE APARTMENTS WILL SUSTAIN MAJOR DAMAGE...INCLUDING SOME WALL AND ROOF FAILURE. HIGH RISE OFFICE AND APARTMENT BUILDINGS WILL SWAY DANGEROUSLY...A FEW TO THE POINT OF TOTAL COLLAPSE. ALL WINDOWS WILL BLOW OUT. AIRBORNE DEBRIS WILL BE WIDESPREAD... AND MAY INCLUDE HEAVY ITEMS SUCH AS HOUSEHOLD APPLIANCES AND EVEN LIGHT VEHICLES. SPORT UTILITY VEHICLES AND LIGHT TRUCKS WILL BE MOVED. THE BLOWN DEBRIS WILL CREATE ADDITIONAL DESTRUCTION. PERSONS...PETS... AND LIVESTOCK EXPOSED TO THE WINDS WILL FACE CERTAIN DEATH IF STRUCK. POWER OUTAGES WILL LAST FOR WEEKS... AS MOST POWER POLES WILL BE DOWN AND TRANSFORMERS DESTROYED. WATER SHORTAGES WILL MAKE HUMAN SUFFERING INCREDIBLE BY MODERN STANDARDS. THE VAST MAJORITY OF NATIVE TREES WILL BE SNAPPED OR UPROOTED. ONLY THE HEARTIEST WILL REMAIN STANDING...BUT BE TOTALLY DEFOLIATED. FEW CROPS WILL REMAIN. LIVESTOCK LEFT EXPOSED TO THE WINDS WILL BE KILLED. AN INLAND HURRICANE WIND WARNING IS ISSUED WHEN SUSTAINED WINDS NEAR HURRICANE FORCE...OR FREQUENT GUSTS AT OR ABOVE HURRICANE FORCE...ARE CERTAIN WITHIN THE NEXT 12 TO 24 HOURS. ONCE TROPICAL STORM AND HURRICANE FORCE WINDS ONSET...DO NOT VENTURE OUTSIDE!

I rushed back to the office to let my family know about the room assignment. They would also be interested in the latest weather reports. It was about one o'clock, and Cecile, Claire, and Paige were already arranging for sleeping accommodations on the floor in my office. Had Cecile been using some of her child and adolescent psychiatry training to calm the kids? The news that we had a real bedroom to sleep in was the first good news they'd had all day. We all left the office to go to the McFarland Building, which adjoined my office building. Paige opened the door to see a spacious room with two double beds, a private bathroom with shower, and a TV. The corner room on the seventh floor had a view of the Superdome, the New Orleans skyline, and the Crescent City Connection spanning the Mississippi River. The only problem was that the two walls of windows might easily blow out in hurricane-force winds. Despite that drawback, it looked a lot more appealing than sleeping on the floor in my office.

We decided to stay.

After we had settled in to the room, I rejoined the group of administrators, nurses, kitchen workers, doctors, and maintenance workers who were transporting the food from the basement to the fourth floor. I had been at Baptist for twenty years, and had never discovered the maze of corridors in the bowels of the hospital basement. The ceramic floors were slippery with condensation near the freezer as we moved out supplies that the chef would use before we lost electricity. The kitchen, pantry, and freezer had tons of food to be moved. As we needed a larger transport vehicle than the hand truck that was available, a nurse wheeled a stretcher into the kitchen, and we piled it high with food. Soon a caravan of stretchers and beds, loaded with food and supplies, shuttled to and from the fourth floor. After we moved most of the perishable food up to safety, I left to check on the status of my group's hospitalized patients.

In addition to my duties as chief of medicine, I also planned to help care for our practice's patients who were in the hospital. My group, Audubon Internal Medicine, would typically have about twenty patients in the hospital. During disasters, many patients would try to get hospitalized in order to be assured of care, should the electricity be lost in their home. Families would sometimes just drop off an elderly relative at the ER doorstep to avoid the inconvenience of taking Grandma along when they evacuated. The dire warnings about Katrina had magnified these trends. Audubon's hospital census had swelled to about thirty patients over the last two days. I called Larry O'Neil, one of the physicians on duty that weekend, to meet with him and assist with rounds. I caught up with him at the nursing station on Five Clara West around two o'clock. His face had not yet lost that youthful glow of a doctor fresh out of training. His brown hair was disheveled, and a large patch over his left eye was held in place by a ragged piece of tape. His green scrubs looked like they had been slept in.

"Larry, what are you doing?" I asked. "What's the matter with your eye?"

"I think my contact is dirty or something. My eye got real red, so I decided to put this patch on it. Don't worry. I'm okay. Really." His speech was even more hurried than usual.

"Well, how are the patients doing? Let me help you see some people."

"I still have four or five patients from yesterday that I've not seen yet. Most of them were consults, but some were admitted through the ER."

"Why didn't you see them yet? What were you doing yesterday afternoon when they came in?" These patients had not been seen for almost twenty-four hours at this point.

"I was home trying to figure out what to do with my cat. I was worrying about my mother-in-law too. What am I going to do with her? I had to spend a long time on the telephone trying to make all the arrangements and getting her taken care of. It took hours! Then I had to decide what to pack to come over here to ride out the hurricane. My poor kitty, she's so confused."

I had my own issues to deal with and had little sympathy for his problems. I was beginning to realize that he might completely unwind in the face of this stress. My partner who was on duty that weekend had asked Larry on Saturday to take over all of his patients so that he could be free to evacuate, having obtained coverage for his patients. Larry had agreed and was now in over his head. I told him that I would round on and care for the unseen patients from yesterday and then check in with him about his progress later.

Fortunately, none of the patients from the day before had any critical problems. Frequent questions from the nursing staff about non-Audubon patients slowed my progress. The nursing staff could not contact many of the physicians, so they asked me about various medical questions popping up with the patients. Now, late on Sunday afternoon, many of the physicians who had come in to round in the morning were gone. The wind outside had steadily increased, and bands of rain were whipping down. Even if a physician could be contacted, a drive to the hospital at this time would have been either extremely dangerous or impossible. The care of their patients fell, by default, on those physicians who remained in the facility. The chairman of medicine was the person whom the nurses ultimately turned to for help when all other avenues failed. With cell phones failing, the staff had difficulty contacting even those physicians who remained in the hospital. The overhead paging system was still operable, but did not extend to the office buildings or the McFarland Building, where many doctors were staying.

By around four o'clock, I finished and caught up with Larry. The eye patch was hanging on by the very last particles of the tape's adhesive. His good eye was glassed over.

"Hey, Richard," he said.

"Hey, Larry. How's it going? Were you able to see the rest of the patients?"

"Almost. I still have some to see on the other side of the hospital."

"Go down and get something to eat. I'll see the rest of them," I told him.

"Okay, where is the food?"

"We moved it to the fourth floor. There should be a serving line set up there. Where are you staying tonight?"

"I'm not sure; maybe I'll just find a place on the floor somewhere."

"Don't do that. Look, you're welcome to stay in our office. It's a lot better than staying in here with these people all strewn about." As evening approached, every common area, hallway, and lobby resembled my teenager's room during a giant sleepover.

"That's a good idea. At least I can put my kitty and other things in there. I don't have a key, though."

"Here you go." I gave him the key. "Bring it back when you're finished. As soon as you can leave tomorrow, get on out of here. Thanks for covering this weekend. I'll take over in the morning."

The wind and rain were now coming continuously. Bands of squalls were pelting the entire area. As dusk prematurely approached around seven o'clock, the street signs bangled in the wind, limbs and branches blew haphazardly down the street, and breezeways howled in protest as gusts blew through. A random mockingbird fought gamely against the force of the storm. Eventually, the frail bird was carried away downwind. Small trees were bending over to the point of snapping. I thought of the room we were in for the evening, with all those windows. By nightfall, the electricity in our part of the city was down, and darkness enveloped the immediate area. The hospital's generator kicked on. The generator supplied electricity for the critical functions in the intensive care units, some minimal lighting in the rest of the facility, and only two elevators.

At the evening crisis meeting, the team reviewed the latest weather reports. Katrina's sustained winds had weakened slightly. The storm surge measured eighteen feet. Katrina would make landfall in the early morning before sunrise as a Category 4 storm. The nursing staff director reported that they would begin moving all patients from their rooms into the hallways if the windows started to blow out. The chef reassured us that the temporary foodservice area on the fourth floor was serving meals and was safe from flooding. Overhead paging, walkie-talkies, beepers, and telephones still provided fairly reliable communications within the hospital. Cell phone service was spotty. An administrator handed me a walkie-talkie before the meeting broke up. The group decided that it would convene again in the morning.

I got a plate of food and went back to see Cecile and the kids in the room. They had scored some food from the vending machine and were munching away. We all could feel the building swaying and shuddering in the winds. In the darkness and rain, the wind screeched as it rounded the corner of the building outside of our room. Should we leave this room in the McFarland Building and go back to my office where it might be safer? We decided to make evacuation plans from the room, should we hear other windows blowing before ours did. The kids cleared a path to the door, in case we needed to escape from flying glass. I told them to pack those things they wanted to bring in a bag near the door, so that we could run out of the room immediately if our windows were the first to go. Our plan was to spring out of the room in no more than thirty seconds, should an emergency strike.

By around ten that night, Cecile and I settled into one of the two queen-size beds, Paige and Claire into the other. I tried to doze off, but the thoughts of the day's events swirled in my mind. How had I arrived in this predicament?

Cecile and I had awakened early Sunday morning, still groggy from the trip from Chapel Hill. The TV and Internet reports from that morning had given us the latest National Hurricane Service forecast. Katrina packed sustained winds greater than 155 miles per hour and was a monster Category 5 hurricane. Urgent pleas by the authorities to evacuate convinced many to leave. Maybe we should have left, too, just after we arrived home.

Even Claire and Paige had awakened much earlier than usual. Instead of arising at the crack of noon, they were up around eight o'clock, preparing for the departure to the hospital. Paige got the digital camera and took more than a hundred pictures of the house, inside and out. The girls made small evacuation bags with two days worth of clothing, anticipating only a short stay at Baptist Hospital. My bag contained an extra shirt, a pair of pants, and boxers. We all packed a small, communal supply of food, which included two bottles of water, some PowerBars, granola bars, apples, a jar of peanut butter, and a sealed pack of pepperoni. I hurriedly secured the outside objects in the yard, which would become flying missiles in a hurricane. Cecile moved the small potted plants inside. We both removed the cypress swing hanging from the hundred-year-old oak tree in the backyard and set it on the ground. Claire walked around the backyard and picked up her tanning equipment—lounge chairs, beach towels, a water bottle, and a mister. Cecile removed from the patio walls all the slates with pictures of French Quarter scenes painted on them. We finished the work on the patio by laying the ping-pong table on the ground so it would not become airborne. Inside, we closed all the drapes and moved the computers away from windows. I thought of the hundreds of thousands of others in the area who were going through a variation of this same drill.

Lastly, the kids got together the animals' cages, food, and bedding. Paige, the animal lover of the family, took charge and packed Angel's bedding and rabbit food. Then she loaded up the food and bowl for Spice, our debonair cat. Maggie, our yellow Lab and the family favorite, followed Paige around as she worked. When Paige put the dog food and bowl in the car, Maggie sensed excitement brewing and began running around in circles near the car.

As we gathered our belongings for the trip, the wind steadily increased. Small branches and twigs began to fall from the water oaks as gusts began to blow. Knowing that we would be in lockdown for a day or two, I decided to take Maggie out for a run. It would give her a chance to release some energy, and me a chance to vent my growing anxiety.

I loaded the kennel into the car. Maggie excitedly jumped about, knowing she would be going to the levee for a run. The short trip to the Mississippi River levee was notable only for the long line of traffic along Jefferson Highway heading out of the city. We weren't caught up in it, but never before had I seen cars backed up as far as I could see on this stretch of highway. Even on the paved top of the levee, cars were illegally traveling upriver to escape the low-lying areas of the city.

Our usual three-mile running route was an out-and-back trip along the grassy batture, a linear, narrow strip of field land and woods between the levee and the water. Maggie had run this route hundreds of times, and it was her absolute favorite activity. But this time, she started lagging behind after making a side trip into the woods after about two miles. I waited for her, but after about another half mile, she could barely walk. I encouraged her to come to me, and we walked together over the top of the levee, near some of the backyards. Then Maggie slumped down, unable to walk whatsoever.

Clearly, she was very ill. Something was seriously wrong. Was she dehydrated? I frantically searched for water in the adjacent backyards. I finally found a hose and a small saucer for a potted plant. I filled it with water and brought it to Maggie. Her tongue was too weak to even lap at the water. She gasped for gulps of the heavy, humid air. I tried to carry her back to the car, but only got several yards. The awkward distribution of her sixty-five pounds prevented me from carrying her any further. I ran back to the car, got the kennel, and brought it to her to use as a carrier. After sliding Maggie into the kennel, I dragged it about a quarter of a mile back to the car, hoisted the kennel in the back, and raced home.

"Maggie's dying!" I yelled as I ran inside our house to get help from Cecile and the kids.

Claire and Paige rushed outside. We pulled Maggie out of the kennel. Her beautiful yellow coat was dirty and matted. Claire called her friend's mom, Dr. Barbie McCord, Maggie's vet. Paige and I got a hose and began hosing her down, thinking that she was overheated. Dr. McCord advised us to get her into an ice bath and give her a shot of steroids, if possible. We carried Maggie in a sheet used as a big sling, up the stairs to the bathtub. Paige and I lifted her into the tub, which was filling with water.

"Shit! She can't even hold up her head." I supported her head so that she would not drown.

"Maggie, you can do it. You can make it," Paige sobbed.

Cecile then walked in to the cramped bathroom and saw the gasping, limp dog in the tub. Her two daughters were crying. All eyes were fixed on the dog's every breath.

"Come on, Maggie," I cried. Maggie's respirations became agonal.

"She's dying. Cecile, she's dying! Look at her breathing," I wailed through my tears. I had seen many patients die in my career. Witnessing the dying experience was never anything I could get used to, and was always an emotional event for me.

All of us were crying uncontrollably as Maggie took her last breath, her head propped up from the rising bathwater in my arms. I turned off the water and opened the drain. We all just waited and sobbed for a few minutes, trying to collect ourselves.

Cecile and I hoisted Maggie's limp, wet body out of the tub and brought her back downstairs to the driveway. While we decided what to do next, Dr. McCord drove up. She and her family were evacuating at this late hour, but she detoured to our house when Claire had called. I was particularly touched by her caring for our dog, despite her concerns about her own safety. She found all of us surrounding Maggie's lifeless body in the driveway.

"I brought a dose of steroids for her," she said.

"Thanks, Barbie. But she just died about five minutes ago. I'm not sure what happened to her. We did the same run we always do."

She took a minute to examine the dead animal before her.

"Maybe she got heatstroke; maybe she got bit by a snake. They can go really fast when that happens. I'm so sorry for you."

"We put her in the ice bath like you said, but she didn't respond."

"There was probably nothing else you could have done."

We stood in the driveway, not knowing what to do or say.

"I can't believe you stopped by," I offered. "You need to get out of here."

"We were getting on the road when you called, and I thought I'd stop by on our way out. I'm not sure where we'll end up."

"Thanks for coming over, Barbie," Cecile said.

We all gave each other hugs. Barbie resumed her evacuation journey to safer ground.

I was still shirtless and sweaty from my run and from bringing Maggie to the car. Cecile and I hauled Maggie to the backyard to bury her near the site where our Siamese cat was buried two years before. I dug a hole as the wind steadily increased. Branches from the trees above fell about us. The approaching storm was not going to deter me. I was giving Maggie a proper burial.

Once a large enough hole was made, I lowered her body into it, sheet and all. Claire, Paige, and Cecile were all around the grave, stunned at the hour's unexpected events. I went inside to write a note to Maggie to toss in her grave with her. The kids went slowly inside to get their bags.

Maggie, you were the best running buddy I ever had. I'll see you later. I tossed the note in the hole and covered the grave. I stood alone next to the mound of freshly shoveled dirt. As I turned to step away, the wind died down for a few moments before the next breeze blew Maggie's spirit away.

A particularly loud gust of wind suddenly came howling around the corner of the McFarland Building. I heard a steady drip, drip, drip inside the room, as water fell from the ceiling onto the metal window ledge. Wind-blown rain was also seeping between the edge of the windows and their frames. The hurricane's noise and my concern over the many windows in the room made sound sleep impossible. I tried to doze, but couldn't stop thinking of the uncontrollable forces at play.

CHAPTER 2

Monday

...you better start swimmin'
Or you'll sink like a stone
For the times they are a-changin'

— Bob Dylan from "The Times They Are
A-Changin'"

"D r. Deichmann, get up," Sean Fowler barked to me over the
phone. "The windows are blowing out all over!" He was
over in the hospital, getting reports from the staff. "The crosswalks
between the buildings are blowing, just like we were worried
about. You can't get over here by the one closest to Napoleon. See
if you can come over by the other one. If you don't get over here
soon, you might be trapped over there in that building and not be
able to get over here to the main campus. We need you over here
now. Get moving."

"Okay. We'll get out of here right away and I'll head on over
as soon as possible," I said. My watch showed 2:13 am.

Everyone else in the room with me was awake. They were all
having a tough time sleeping anyway.

"Let's go," I said. "We need to get out of here now. The windows are starting to blow around the hospital and crosswalks. Get your bags and let's hurry over to my office."

We darted for our bags, as per the drill just a few hours before, and fled the room in seconds. The faint light from the generator power cast a twilight into the hallway. The elevators were out, so we took the steps from the seventh floor to the second floor, so that we could cross over to my office. The stairwell was completely black, except for the steady light of our flashlights. We walked over to the Napoleon Medical Plaza building, and then up its darkened stairwell to the eighth floor. Cecile, Paige, and Claire set up pads and pillows in an interior hallway of the office. They closed all the doors to offices leading to exterior windows. Satisfied that they were safe, I retraced my path by flashlight back down the stairs to the second floor.

I made my way back to the crosswalk over Clara Street, connecting the McFarland Building to the hospital. The previously enclosed crosswalk now had glass flying all over the inside of the walkway. The wind was slamming through it unimpeded. Part of the ceiling had collapsed, and ceiling tiles flew around, shattering into pieces as they collided into the walls or floors. It was too dangerous to even survey the damage, much less try to run the gauntlet through the walkway. I hurried to the crosswalk connecting the garage to the hospital, now worried that there would be no way for me to get across, since that was the only remaining access to the hospital. The second crosswalk was still intact, but the whole structure was shaking so violently that it could become impassable at any second. I sprinted across the thirty-yard hallway to the hospital, praying that one of the massive windows would not shatter just as I passed. My prayers were answered, and I went straight to the command center.

Sean, Susan, and several other key personnel were in the fourth-floor command center. The weather reports indicated Katrina was nearing landfall. It was still a hundred miles away from us. How much worse would things get as it got closer? Water was already filling the streets. Three feet of water now blocked any escape from the parking garage. Internet reports indicated widespread flooding was occurring throughout the area. The sky outside was pitch black. Sheets of rain pelted the windows, only reaching the ground after flowing down the building's walls. No one dared stare out of a window for any length of time, for fear the wind might shatter the glass inches from one's face. The morning light would arrive in just about two hours and allow a clearer, firsthand view of the damage so far.

The damage reports from inside the hospital included not only the crosswalk problems, but also windows blowing out throughout the hospital. Almost all of the windows in the Medical Intensive Care Unit had shattered; windows in some of the regular, acute-care rooms were gone; and several massive windows in the lobby areas were blown out. After hearing the reports, I decided to wander around, to see for myself what was happening.

The hallways were packed with hundreds of people lying on the floors. Many of them had moved to safer hallway areas. Their previous campsites had become unsafe from flying shards of glass blowing about or from water dripping down from the ceiling. Security personnel roped off the dangerous areas, but they could do little to stop the wind and rain from roaring through some of the common areas. Some evacuees were listening to music, others talking, a few praying. I got the sense that almost all of them thought that they had outsmarted the storm by finding refuge in the sturdy hospital. If Katrina could do this to Baptist, what kind of chance would they have had in their own small, wooden homes?

The eighth-floor Medical Intensive Care Unit was covered with glass. The nurses had swept the chunks of glass back into the rooms and closed the doors to the wind and rain. This unit was the place where the sickest patients in the hospital were cared for. Complicated post-operative patients and very ill non-surgical patients were admitted to this unit, to be monitored closely by nurses and high-tech equipment. All the patients here were critically ill, and several were on ventilators. The nurses had moved them out of their windowed rooms to the safer common areas in the unit. The scene was unlike any I had witnessed in any intensive care unit I had ever stepped into. A critically ill patient needs physical space to accommodate all of the high-tech support equipment. Typically, these technologies include several intravenous bags, intravenous pumps, a heart monitor with its telemetry leads, a blood pressure monitor, a central venous catheter, a Foley catheter, and a mechanical ventilator with all of its wires and tubing. The patients in the unit now were cramped in the common areas right next to each other. The beeping of their alarms, pumps, and ventilators, mixed with the patients' groans and breaths, made for a hellish cacophony.

I checked on a couple of the patients who were having trouble breathing. I made some minor adjustments to their therapies and answered questions from the nurses. None of the patients had any immediate life-threatening complications, and they were stable on their current medical therapies. I left and took the lone working elevator back to the fourth floor, hanging out at the command center until daybreak.

As dawn broke, the full force of the storm was hitting. Whitecaps blew off the tops of the waves in the streets. Pieces of roofs crashed into the buildings and clunked down into the water. Trees and telephone poles toppled over. Sheet metal shrieked as it ripped away from the building, flying through the air and crashing into the immovable structures still standing. The wind had finally reached its maximum intensity after almost twenty-four hours.

The wind then changed direction and began to diminish. I needed to get back over to see how my family was doing. The only passable crosswalk to my office now had several windows blown out. Glass was not flying through it, so I raced back across to the office building. I sprinted up the stairway to the eighth floor to see Cecile and my two girls.

"Dad, come see this!" Paige insisted.

She led me to one of the windows with a postcard view of the downtown skyline. The roof of the Superdome had blown off! The smooth white dome was peeled off like an onion, exposing the roof's ragged black under-structure. Parts of the roof flapped in the breeze. My eyes stayed glued to the scene in disbelief.

Cecile, Claire, and Paige wanted to get out of the office. Cabin fever was setting in. I didn't want them to risk the danger of going back to the hospital through the crosswalk. So instead, we went outside to the parking garage, so everyone could see what Katrina had wrought.

We avoided getting too close to the edge of the garage, for fear that flying debris might strafe us. The wind was still around fifty miles per hour. Whitecaps danced in the street. Paige leaned her thin body into the wind. In every direction, trees were snapped, power lines were down, and debris blew through the flooded streets. Paige took a few pictures, and we returned to the office until Katrina finally blew herself out.

I went over to the hospital and we had another meeting at the command center. Eric Yancovich was in charge of the physical plant and a master at the designing, building, and repairing of the sprawling hospital complex. Eric's big shoulders, thick neck, and barrel chest rivaled those of many football players I know. Dave Goodson was René's right-hand man, whom he had personally picked to tackle the really tough problems no one else in the administration could solve. His boyish face, short haircut, and squeaky-clean look complemented his positive, can-do attitude. Eric and Dave gave a preliminary summary of the damage to the hospital. The hospital was still on generator power, so only two elevators in the facility were functional. The stairways were lit, and provided the fastest, most reliable means of transportation between floors. In addition to the windows being blown out in many locations, the crosswalk connecting the McFarland Building and the hospital had sustained structural damage and was unsafe to walk across. Water was leaking from the ceilings of most of the upper floors due to roof leaks. Rainwater seeping in through the broken windows on other floors produced ceiling leaks on the lower floors. Soggy carpets throughout the facility made a squishy sound when stepped upon. Eric's team had boarded up all the windows in the intensive care unit and had roped off other areas that were unsafe.

The chef had served thousands of meals over the last twenty-four hours. Anticipating that the three feet of water in the streets would recede shortly, he planned to partially resume operations downstairs in the basement later in the day. Since the basement was below street level, as long as water accumulated in the street, the basement could begin flooding. He expected that the street flooding would recede by Tuesday. Once that happened, he planned to begin transporting the food back downstairs.

The hospital security department had finally gotten a fairly firm fix on how many people were in the facilities. More than two thousand people were in the hospital, including the more than two hundred patients. Hundreds of pets—dogs, cats, rabbits, even a ferret—had been carried in too. Initially, a kennel space was created in the medical records department. The number of animals had grown to the point where the kennel area was overwhelmed, and it had been relocated outside to the Magnolia parking garage. Owners could visit with their animals and walk them in the garage. The security personnel reported that animals were also roaming about the hospital. They were making efforts to keep all the animals outside.

A nursing supervisor reported on the status of the various nursing units. The hundreds of people littered about the hallways slowed their patient care. Additionally, requests and questions from the many non-patients in the hospital were sucking up their time. Having only two functioning elevators and no pneumatic tube system made it difficult to transport supplies and medications to the nursing stations around the hospital. Nurses had trouble contacting the patients' physicians, further compromising care. The nursing supervisor's comments hit home, because the night before, I cared for a patient when the nurses couldn't contact the patient's physician.

The patient was on the fifth floor and had become suddenly short of breath during the night. The patient had undergone a total hip replacement surgery several days before. None of the patient's physicians were available. A nurse called me to evaluate the patient, an elderly, quiet lady named Mrs. Gautreaux.

"Mrs. Gautreaux, I'm Doctor Deichmann," I said. "How are you feeling?"

"Oh, just fine," she said as her chest heaved up and down.

"It looks like you're pretty short of breath with all that heavy breathing." I counted her breaths per minute.

"Yeah, I am kind of short of breath. I'll be fine with a little oxygen though, Doc."

"Mrs. Gautreaux, your doctor's not here now, so is it okay if I take care of you for now? I'll need to examine you first."

"Is it okay? Sure, it's okay. I really appreciate you being here."

I found that she had a rapid heart rate of 120 and a relatively low blood pressure. She was breathing twenty-six times per minute. Her lungs sounded clear. Her heart exam revealed no murmurs or abnormal beats. The hip wound didn't appear infected, and her legs had no swelling. A small, battery-powered device showed that the oxygen saturation in her blood was 88 percent. It should have been around 98 percent. The clinical setting suggested a pulmonary embolus, a life-threatening condition in which a blood clot breaks off from a vein in the leg and lodges in the lung. The problem is a well-known complication of hip surgery.

The suspicion of such a diagnosis would usually set off a chain of events, including sophisticated radiology studies, blood tests, and a blood gas test, which is a precise measurement of the amount of oxygen in the blood. A respiratory therapist would be called to perform the blood gas and to make adjustments in the supplemental oxygen she was receiving by a nasal cannula. The pharmacist would be contacted, and blood-thinning medication would be sent up immediately. The hospital had very few of its usual processes in place. None of these diagnostic tests was available at the time. I decided to treat the patient empirically with a type of blood-thinning medication which did not require a lot of laboratory follow-up or intravenous pumps. The nurse gave her the first dose of the injection and increased her oxygen. I told the patient to let the nurse know if she started to feel more short of breath. I promised her that I'd check on her later, and left the unit.

I refocused on the meeting, and everyone seemed to be giving a story about our communications problems. Cell phones weren't working, and the hospital overhead paging system was out now. The telephones and beepers still mostly worked, but not everywhere. E-mail was fairly reliable. I began to think of how we might develop some improvised system of caring for the patients who no longer had a physician on site or available by phone.

The administration requested that the medical staff try to discharge patients from their active inpatient status, if possible. Although the patients could not leave the hospital at the time, at least they would not be consuming the limited resources of the nursing staff, dietary staff, pharmacy, and housekeeping. Such a status would also allow for these patients to leave the hospital more quickly when conditions did improve.

When it was time for my report, I again brought up the poor communications impairing the ability of nurses to contact physicians. I reported how nurses tried unsuccessfully to get in touch with physicians who were covering for their partners. The nurses found it practically impossible to figure out which physicians were covering for each other, and for which patients. They could not reach most of the physicians. I had come up with a plan.

I assigned a staff physician to be the doctor in charge of each nursing unit and the intensive care unit. This physician would be responsible for the patients on that unit, even though the physician may not be those patients' attending physician. The physician in charge would let the nurses know how to contact him or her, and the assignment list would be available at each nursing unit. The twenty to thirty physicians present also would continue seeing their own patients and caring for them. Finally, I supported the administration's request that patients be discharged, if possible, to the general population, in order to decrease the already-heavy demands on the hospital and nursing resources.

The meeting broke up, and the physicians went to their new assignments. I got to work checking on my group's thirty to thirty-five patients. Larry was off now and needed the down time. As I made my hospital rounds, I noticed that the new system of nursing unit physician assignments was working well in providing an authority in charge of patient care, someone who was both reliable and available.

Mrs. Gautreaux's nurse stopped me to give me her report. The patient's breathing, heart rate, and blood pressure had returned to normal. The nurse had administered two doses of the blood-thinning medicine so far, and the patient had not developed any new complaints. I went in to see her.

"How are you feeling this morning, Mrs. Gautreaux?" I asked her.

"I'm fine," she said. "But it sure was hard to sleep with all that racket going on outside. Then they came and moved me into the hall in the middle of the night."

"The nurses were worried the window in your room might break in the storm. You're back in your room now, though."

"Yeah, but when am I getting something to eat? I'm starving."

"The hurricane's disrupted a lot of the usual way we do things," I said, stating the obvious. "But I'll ask the staff to send for a tray for you."

I listened to her heart and lungs, and found her physical exam unremarkable. After reassuring her that I thought she would be okay, I left to continue rounds.

The disruptions in normal procedures extended to every facet of hospital care. The laboratory and radiology departments offered only limited services. The usual mechanisms to transport patients to different areas of the hospital had broken down, since few elevators worked and few transport workers were available. The operating rooms had no lights.

As in Mrs. Gautreaux's case, adequate care could be improvised. But Katrina had blown away any sophisticated care involving high-tech diagnostic tests, consultants, surgery, or complicated medical treatments.

I went down to the third floor, which housed mostly cancer patients. One of our group's patients, Mrs. Emma Washington, was hospitalized when her lung cancer caused her to develop pneumonia. I knocked on her door and went in to see her.

"Good morning, Mrs. Washington. How are you doing today?" I asked.

She was an elderly lady who also suffered from Alzheimer's disease, high blood pressure, and bad back pain from arthritis. Her memory loss caused her to rely on her husband to do most of the talking for her. Mr. Washington stood alongside her bed in his starched brown pants and white shirt. His brown coat hung on the back of the chair he had slept in at her side last night.

"Earl, tell the doctor," she muttered in his direction.

"She be doing just fine, Doc," he said. "We be wanting to get out of here and go back home where I can take care of her."

"Is she coughing any more?" I asked him.

"No. She be breathing fine and sleeping fine. Can we go home now?"

I listened to her lungs and didn't hear any of the typical crackling sounds of pneumonia.

"Well, I agree with you. She does sound good. I think she's clearing up that pneumonia. The only problem is there's a hurricane still passing by. You can't leave yet; it's too dangerous. Y'all should be able to leave by tomorrow, though."

"Okay. I just want to get Emma home as soon as possible," he said.

"See you tomorrow," I said, and left to finish rounds. At that point, I assumed they still had a home.

As Monday afternoon approached, a general sense of relief settled in among everyone. The hospital and staff had made it through the worst of Katrina. The sky became a welcome shade of blue, and the wind decreased to a pleasant, stiff breeze. The water in the street was quickly receding. By six o'clock that evening, the streets outside the hospital were dry.

Some evacuees decided to head out for home as dusk approached. A few physicians left, and I encouraged Dr. O'Neil to leave too. But given the lack of electricity in the outside world, he and almost all of the evacuees decided to stay for the night and set out in the morning.

After I finished seeing my group's patients late in the afternoon, I tracked down the rest of the Deichmann clan. They were wandering around, taking in the unusual sights, both inside and outside of the hospital. I finally found them on the second floor near a food line, where they had scored some apples, chips, and soft drinks.

"Dickie, what do you think about trying to get back home tonight?" Cecile asked hopefully.

"The roads look dry. Let's go see the house!" Claire chirped.

"Come on, Dad," Paige added.

"Let's check it out, gang," I said.

Paige and Claire were gloating over the fact that they would probably be missing another day of school as the car pulled out of the Baptist parking garage Monday evening. The journey home was immediately complicated by fallen trees, house siding, fallen telephone poles, and downed power lines. As twilight beckoned, the winds steadily lessened and the clouds cleared. Many nearby homes had missing roofs, accordion-like fences partially blown down, and yards filled with debris. Nearby, a two-story home had collapsed and crushed the first story and its contents. House siding and shrubbery littered the yards, streets, and sidewalks. As we proceeded down Claiborne Avenue, rivulets of water, which had not yet receded, blocked the way and flowed across the roadway. Massive geysers mysteriously shot up from the manholes, reaching ten feet into the sky.

After several futile attempts to ford the streams with the SUV, Cecile and I decided to turn back and head for the safety of the medical center once again. We knew that we had weathered a wicked, howling hurricane, and this would be our last night sleeping on the floor of a hot office building. The air conditioning had shut off when the generators kicked on almost twenty-four hours ago. None of the windows in any of the buildings could be opened, and the temperature was steadily rising throughout the facility. By tomorrow, the water would have receded, the debris would be removed, and passage home was almost assured. A city where Mardi Gras clean-up crews can tidy up the trash after a parade within fifteen minutes would surely have the way home passable after another twelve hours, or so I thought.

Once we returned to the hospital, I picked up the one allotted serving of food reserved for the staff. I brought it to the rest of the family in my office on the eighth floor, which was getting uncomfortably warm. We laughed and joked as we enjoyed our last meal in our first-ever evacuation shelter. The kids wolfed down the serving of spaghetti and some french bread, while Cecile and I settled for a couple of apples and granola bars that had been packed from home.

Tomorrow would bring the comforts of home again. Tomorrow would bring a pantry full of food and the soft familiarity of our own beds. Tomorrow we would put the inconvenience of Katrina behind us and get back to our usual routine.

Or so we thought.

CHAPTER 3

Tuesday

Water broke past the levee
My heart beats hard and heavy

— Cowboy Mouth from "On the Avenue"

"Dad, let's go," Paige said. "Let's see what the house looks like." She was packed and ready to go. Sunlight streaked over the treetops outside.

Claire, normally not one to voluntarily get up before eight in the morning, had already brushed her hair and gotten the rabbit cage ready for the trip home.

"Look, before y'all leave, you need to clean up the mess the rabbit's made in that exam room," I said. "Check out the kitty litter box too. There's a mess around it. Then I'll bring the animals to the car and we'll leave."

"I can't wait to get back to my house. What do you think it'll be like?" Cecile asked to no one in particular. "I hope we didn't get any trees through the roof. I guess we'll find out soon."

Our plan was to go home and survey the damage. If the place was livable, I would drop everyone off and head back over to the hospital. If it was too badly damaged, we would make whatever repairs we could and come back to my office. One way or another, Spice the cat and Angel the rabbit would be staying home. They had been cooped up for two days and were going crazy.

We drove out of the garage onto the dry streets around the hospital as the morning dew glistened on the surrounding grass. Telephone poles, wires, and oak tree limbs still littered the streets, making the going slow. The unexpected presence of a creek rushing across Claiborne Avenue near Ursuline Academy made passage impossible. We turned back toward the hospital and tried to outflank the unanticipated waterway. Eventually, we found that water blocked all the routes leading toward our home in River Ridge. The canal along Washington Avenue led to the Seventeenth Street Canal and then into Lake Pontchartrain. The water there had risen to an inch from the top of the cement barrier along the canal walls. Angry water rushed through it, exerting a massive force on the feeble cement barrier. The water level was about three feet above the car. A break or even a small shift of the ten-inch-thick cement barriers would dump millions of gallons of water onto our small SUV immediately. I turned to Cecile.

"C., it's too dangerous to be driving next to this thing," I said.

"No kidding. Let's get out of here. What's plan B?" she said.

"We can make it!" Claire complained. "Don't give up. I don't want to go back to your office."

"We've been trying, but it's no use," I said. After thirty to forty minutes of testing all avenues of escape, the furthest we had traveled from the hospital in any one direction was about a mile and a half.

We developed Plan B. Cecile's mother Anne and stepfather Carroll lived only about a mile from the hospital. Maybe we could make it to her house and check on them. They had decided to ride out the storm as usual. Their hundred-year-old elevated home in uptown New Orleans had weathered a century of hurricanes.

They felt perfectly secure from the threat of winds and floods. Besides, now in their eighties, an evacuation for them was no easy undertaking. If we could get to their house on Valmont Street, anyone who wanted could stay there. The rabbit and cat would stay for sure. I'd visit the in-laws for a little while and then head back to the hospital.

As the sun came up over the remaining treetops, we dodged the limbs, trees, and power lines on our way to their house. We saw whole houses collapsed, a maple tree snapped in two, and large swaths of roofing in the roads. Sometimes the only passage was over the grassy neutral ground between roads or through someone's mangled yard.

The streams flowing through many of the streets puzzled us. The rain had stopped more than twelve hours ago. Why was there still so much water in unusual places? The radio reported vague, unconfirmed stories that one or more levees had broken. But what parts of the city were affected? Was it serious? When were they going to plug up the breaks? How bad were the holes in the levees? What was the best way to get out now? The radio provided no reliable answers or guidance.

Cell phones were still not working, and we arrived unannounced at Anne and Carroll's house. Cecile knocked on the door, not knowing what to expect. The door eventually swung open.

"Oh my goodness. I'm so glad to see you!" Anne said as she opened the door for her daughter. "Look, Carroll, Cecile's here!" Anne yelled back into the darkened house.

"Mom, are you okay? I'm so glad to see you too!" Cecile hugged her and finally stepped inside. The rest of us followed after, exchanging hugs and kisses. Cecile walked into the living room and eyed the worn-out rugs, the antique sideboard, and the general state of mild disrepair that accompanies an aging home. Her mother and stepfather were fixtures in that home, always reluctant to leave.

"Mom, did y'all do okay? How much damage did you get?"

"We did pretty well. Some water came in from a broken window, and we had some roof damage. It looks like we lost a couple of shutters too. We were lucky. Across the street, you saw how the tree fell on their house?"

"Can I get anyone a bloody mary?" Carroll offered. "We still have some ice."

"Oh, man. How I would enjoy one of those. Maybe it would help settle my nerves," I said. "I better not, though. I'm gonna need to go back to the hospital."

"We've heard the levees have broken," Anne explained. "But it looks like we'll probably stay. The guy next door has a generator and he said he's staying. We can get what we need from him."

The radio reports hinted that the only available route out of the city now was across the Crescent City Connection, the bridge over the Mississippi River.

"I think maybe we should go," Cecile said. "Mom, you really ought to go, too. The levees have broken. The city's filling up with water. You may not be able to escape later." Cecile tried to convince herself—as much as her mother—of the need to leave. "I don't know if I can leave you here. The water's coming up quickly. We don't have much time to decide. What will you do here with no electricity?"

"We'll be okay," Anne said.

Cecile turned toward me next and connected eye to eye.

"What if I get stranded while trying to escape with the kids? Why won't you come with us?" she demanded of me.

"I just feel like they really need me at the hospital," I said, knowing that my family really needed me too.

"What to do with the rabbit?" she asked. "Which car to take? Where am I going to get gas? I don't know what to do." Major decisions were not Cecile's forte.

She turned to her younger daughter. "Paige, what do you think we should do?"

"Let's go," Paige said firmly.

"How about you, Claire?"

"I don't care. I don't know what's best," Claire punted back.

Cecile turned to me again. "We're leaving. Are you coming?" It was a challenge as much as a question.

My mind now raced with anxiety, as a new set of fears attacked. Was it a good idea for us to separate? How exactly was Cecile going to escape? What if she got trapped by rising water before getting out of town? Did she have enough gas to get to Lafayette, the home of our friends she would be trying to reach? There would be no way for her to communicate, should trouble occur. No one knew how far it was to the next working gas station. What were the alternatives if she stayed at the hospital with me? How could I leave my responsibilities to the patients? How could I leave my responsibilities to my own family?

I had confidence in Cecile that somehow she could make it to safety with the kids. I knew I'd be needed more at the hospital.

"I'm going to stay," I said.

Since Anne and Carroll decided to stay, they agreed to keep Angel with them. We set up her rabbit cage under the raised house in the shade and supplied her with plenty of food and water. Spice the cat stayed in the car for the planned escape from the flooding city.

Since time to leave the city was running out as the seconds ticked away, we hurried back to the hospital garage, dodging debris along the way. The plan was for Cecile and the kids to pack up the SUV with some food and water from my office. Since both of our cars only had a half a tank of gas, I would siphon gas from one of the cars to the SUV, the designated escape vehicle.

I had not siphoned gas since I was a kid. Back then, the plastic tubing of my jump rope worked perfectly in transferring gas from the car gas tank to the push lawn mower I used to cut the grass. Where could I get the right size tubing now? I thought that maybe the tubing used to deliver oxygen by a nasal cannula might work. I tracked down a respiratory tech who found several lengths of tubing which we connected together. I brought the tubing to the cars, which Cecile had parked gas tank to gas tank. The flexible tubing kept bending upon itself after going only a short distance into the donor gas tank. Finally, after making several passes and wiggling the tubing gently, the tip seemed to be in the pool of gasoline at the bottom of the tank. I began sucking on the other end and immediately became light-headed and dizzy. Lungfuls of the vapors shot straight to my head. I was getting sicker and sicker. Despite my efforts, only vapors would come out of the tubing. Convinced I was suffering irreversible brain damage from this futile exercise, I decided Cecile was going to have to take her chances on less than half a tank of gas. Out of options, she promised to fill up the tank at the first gas station.

Claire and Paige loaded themselves and Spice the cat into the car after giving me a hug. They were in a hurry to leave. They didn't want to waste any more time going back to the room in the McFarland Building that they had stayed in on Sunday evening, to retrieve a few of their belongings left behind in the rush to escape that night. I gave Cecile a long hug. Neither was at all sure what was about to happen to us. As she drove off, a heaviness welled up inside of me. The sensation filled my chest and mushroomed upward into my throat. I lowered my head and walked half-heartedly back to the hospital.

The previously optimistic reports of food supplies led me to believe that at least everyone would have plenty of food and water at the hospital. On my way to the morning crisis meeting at ten AM, I passed by the food line to get some breakfast. When I was served a breakfast of grits, scrambled eggs, and a sausage in a ten-ounce Styrofoam cup, I knew that we could be in trouble if this type of rationing was necessary already.

Shortly before the meeting, René came to talk with me. His Cajun ancestors had never had to deal with this type of catastrophe. The hospital couldn't care for the more than two thousand people in the facility. He had received reports that the entire city was going to flood shortly because of multiple breaks in the levees. The hospital generators could fail if the water got too high. He had made the decision to evacuate the facility. He asked for my help in the enormous mission ahead.

The decision caught me unsuspecting, but only because events were spinning out of control faster than I could process them. Since its founding in 1925, the 350-bed hospital had never been evacuated. Such an undertaking, particularly under the current conditions, would be a massive effort. The admission that Mother Baptist was not up to the task of protecting the community hit me hard. I felt a personal failure in being unable to perform the task of the hospital to care for the community in its time of need. These were dire times. I would refocus my service to evacuating the thousands of people here to safety.

I agreed wholeheartedly with the decision to evacuate, and pledged my support. If floodwaters knocked out the electricity in the city for an extended period of time, the hospital could not function effectively on generator power alone indefinitely. Even if the generators continued to work, they did not supply air conditioning. The inside was becoming more and more stifling because of the loss of the cooling system since Sunday night, two days ago. If we did lose the generators, patients would clearly be at much greater risk by staying here. All lights, elevators, and refrigerators would be out. The minimal communications working now would be out. Running water would most likely stop. If the city did flood, we could not easily re-supply ourselves, which would quickly become necessary, since we were already depleting our stores of food and water. Food was already being rationed in the overcrowded facility.

At the disaster meeting, we discussed the strategy for evacuation. With the medical staff in attendance, I directed that the staff use a triage system to evacuate the sickest patients first. This first group to evacuate would be the intensive care unit patients, the neonatal intensive care unit patients, and high-risk obstetric patients. The physicians in charge of the various nursing units would medically evaluate the patients on their units and evacuate them according to the severity of their condition. The "do not resuscitate" patients were given the lowest priority. These DNR patients would continue to be cared for, but would be evacuated after the rest of the patients. Dr. Horace Baltz, an internist who had been on the staff longer than anyone around, recommended that we no longer see our own private patients, and that we allow the doctor in charge of that particular nursing unit to assume the medical care of all the patients on that unit. All the physicians present agreed with this idea so that no duplication of work would be necessary.

Even though the plan called for evacuation, no one knew exactly who was coming to get us. Soon the water might be too high for us to drive out of the garage. We assumed that the National Guard would come to help, since there was a contingent of National Guard troops who had taken up refuge in the hospital along with everyone else.

Meanwhile, some supplies and food had already been sent back down to the basement when the hurricane had passed and it appeared the worst was over. Now squads of people were needed to haul the equipment, food, water, and supplies back upstairs again. The administration began arranging for other facilities to accept the Baptist patients. The closest hospital facilities capable of accepting patients were at least sixty miles away, making for a logistical nightmare in transporting patients that far.

The doctors left the meeting charged with the knowledge that we were participating in a historic event. Our calling was to save lives. The opportunity to save thousands of lives was not only humbling but also invigorating. The staff had never planned for or even envisioned such an event. The hospital had practiced disaster drills, but never a facility-wide evacuation.

Shortly after we left the meeting around eleven, the streets began to fill with water. The water started as a dribble coming from Clara Street. The timid little trickle stayed in the gutter along the side of the street as it disappeared into the large drain in front of us. After only two or three minutes, the drain refused to swallow the enlarging stream of water racing to its opening. The water pooled at the mouth of the drain as simultaneous new streams came toward us from the other two directions. Within a couple of minutes, the streams had turned into rivulets similar to the ones I had seen earlier in the day. With nowhere to drain, the water bridged the street from gutter to gutter. From then on, it was only a matter of how high it would get. Within two hours, the streets were totally impassable. Escape by car out of the garage was out of the question now. We were trapped and at the mercy of others to save us.

Dr. Bill Armington, a radiologist specializing in brain imaging, caught up with me outside the crisis center after I had seen enough of the ongoing flooding.

"Hey, Richard, I found a secret passage to the helipad," he said with a sly look on his face.

"What are you talking about?" I asked. "That thing hasn't been used in fifteen years."

"Come on. We need to do some hiking. It's a long way up to get to it. But you can do it, you're a triathlete. Bring your flashlight."

He brought me to an area on the second floor of the hospital that had a stairwell connecting it to a separate stairwell in the Magnolia parking garage. We walked down to the base of the first stairwell, crossed over to the Magnolia parking garage stairwell, and then hiked up the nine floors of the building with flashlights lighting the way. Bill himself was a good athlete who had hiked a number of mountain ranges. Handling the twenty-two flights of stairs to the helipad was just a warm-up exercise for him. Once we climbed to the top, we walked across a pebbled, blacktopped roof to an area underneath the helipad. The helipad was perched on steel beams like flamingo legs. Bill and I walked up the final four flights of steel stairs until we were standing on the top of the structure, high above any of the surrounding buildings. From one side of the helipad, a covered catwalk sloped downward toward the stairwell.

"What a view," I commented. The 360-degree view afforded an unobstructed panorama of the entire city.

"Hey, there's a helicopter," Bill said, pointing off in the distance.

"You think this thing is sturdy enough for choppers to land on?" I wondered aloud.

"It better be. We'll need it."

"They did some type of work on it awhile ago to bring it up to working order again, but I'm not sure if it was finished. This thing hasn't been used in ten or fifteen years."

"We'll be testing it soon," Bill said as we continued to enjoy the view.

"Let's go back down and start getting patients ready to evacuate from this thing," I said.

Bill led me back by a different route. We walked down a circular ramp used by cars to enter the various levels of the Magnolia parking garage, until we got to the second parking level. A crawlspace just big enough for one person to get through led back into the electrical room on the second floor of the hospital.

By the time we got back into the hospital, a National Guard truck had pulled up to the hospital emergency room loading ramp, and people were being loaded onto the truck bed. The ramp's one end connected to the street, now flooded in the knee-deep water. The other end gradually rose out of the water up to the first floor, where the ER was located. Since the truck was not evacuating people to another hospital, sick patients could not be transported. The fifteen people who got on the truck were all ambulatory and could take care of themselves. As the Guard left with the first load of evacuees, they assured us that more trucks were on the way, and that soon they would have the whole facility evacuated to safety. The staff and patients who remained cheered the truck as it left. They thought they were next.

Hope steadily faded as the water continued to inch higher. A second National Guard truck attempted to reach the hospital but stalled out in the water about four blocks from the hospital. We could spot the immobilized vehicle from the upper floors. So ended any possibility of a land-based evacuation route.

Susan, the disaster commander, was trying to contact the surrounding hospitals to arrange for transfer of the patients by helicopter to their facilities. All cell phones and most telephones were out, and it was very difficult to communicate with the other facilities. Internet communications and e-mail were working, to some degree. The smattering of National Guard troops and New Orleans Police Department (NOPD) officers in the hospital had radios, which allowed the staff to contact some outside facilities more effectively.

Dozens of people crowded around the exits from the hospital. The lobby on Clara Street was filled with more than a hundred people, looking helplessly at the rising water. The morning's early promise of evacuating with the help of the National Guard trucks turned out to be a heartbreaker. The crowd on the ER loading ramp stayed on long after it was clear that no more land vehicles would be arriving. Smaller groups in the parking garages across the street gazed hopelessly over the waist-high concrete walls from the different parking levels. I felt like I was part of a group of shipwrecked castaways on a deserted island, hoping someone, somewhere, would eventually find us.

Out of the crowd in the lobby, Earl and Emma Washington emerged, making their way in a distinguished fashion toward the outside steps leading down to the water.

"Excuse me, excuse me, please," Mr. Washington said. He was leading his wife by the hand to the steps.

"Wait! Where are you going?" a nurse asked.

"My wife and I are going home."

"Well, how are you gonna get there? It's flooded."

"We just gonna walk and take it slow, honey." He started descending the steps.

"No," she pleaded. "Don't."

"Listen, baby, I've seen a lot worse things than this in my life. I need to get to my home, where I can be taking care of my Emma. We gotta get outta here any way we can."

His gait was slow and deliberate as he stepped down each of the steps leading into the water. He and his wife slowly entered the ever-deepening lake outside the hospital. Mr. Washington led the way in his dark brown suit and his beige felt hat. His wife followed, clutching his hand, in a light green dress which she tried to raise to keep it dry. With each step down, the water rose higher. When they reached the bottom, the water washed up to their waists. They proceeded across the area that once was the sidewalk until they stepped down onto the street. By now, the water was up to his chest and lapping against her breasts.

Their pace slowed as a hundred people looked at the spectacle in amazement, but the Washingtons never looked back. They seemed to be preparing for a fundamentalist baptism ceremony, in which the initiates dress in their Sunday best, walk into the river, and become totally submerged as they give themselves to the Lord. After about thirty yards, each step was precarious, their feet not knowing what surface, if any, they would find. Eventually, their progress stopped and they just stood there. The nurse who asked them not to go then waded down the steps and into the water to help them.

"I'm coming. Don't worry, Mr. Washington," she called.

He had a puzzled look on his face, as if he suddenly realized he wouldn't be walking home after all. The nurse reached them and cradled their arms inside her own. They slowly cruised back to the steps.

No one was getting out of here on foot.

Word from the walkie-talkie on my belt indicated that helicopters might be arriving, and that patients in the ICU were being mobilized for transport to the helipad. I hurried up to the helipad to evaluate the situation.

Along the way, I ran into Dr. John Skinner, the head of the pathology department at the hospital. He was a tall, lanky, bespectacled man in his fifties. His deep voice and trimmed beard gave him the air of a college professor. Among his many duties, he was the director of the hospital morgue. The morgue was located in the basement, now about ten feet under water.

"John, I need to talk with you about some things," I said.

"Sure, what is it?" he said.

"What's the deal with the morgue now?"

"Well, it's obviously totally submerged and without electricity. We have a number of bodies in the refrigerator down there, all of which are under water."

"How many bodies do you think are stored there now?"

"I'm pretty sure we have nine. The funeral homes stopped coming to pick up the bodies two or three days before the storm hit."

"Boy, that's going to be a mess when the water goes down." I couldn't imagine the stench.

"Yes, it definitely will be."

"What are we going to do with any new bodies?" Baptist would usually have about one death a day, given the many geriatric and cancer patients who were cared for at the facility. In these conditions, even more deaths would be likely.

"We've already had two DNR patients expire since it flooded on Sunday night," he informed me.

"So where are you putting the bodies?"

"We decided to set up a morgue in the chapel. It's out of the way and can be secured easily."

"Okay. Keep in touch with me about the number of bodies you're keeping there."

We continued on our separate ways. But as I made the long trip back up to the helipad, I couldn't shake the image of the chapel being used as a morgue. The hospital chapel was a place I had gone to pray on occasion. Double wooden doors welcomed visitors with the single word, "CHAPEL." The small room had a tasteful altar, always decorated with flowers. About eight wooden pews faced the altar for sitting or kneeling. A small stained-glass window in shades of yellow and white added to the spiritual atmosphere. Now the pews had corpses lying on them. In a way, I guess it made sense. No matter how much sense it made, though, I knew I could never again think of the chapel in the same way.

I finally hiked back up to the helipad. A few people milled about on the pad itself and inside the fifty-foot catwalk connecting the pad with the Magnolia garage stairwell. The helipad had no railing around it and nothing to prevent a fall off its edge. If someone did fall, a three-foot horizontal section of chain-link fencing surrounding the pad might catch the person before falling to an instant death far below. I radioed to the ICU to send up a patient and tried to begin organizing the deck. We needed water, oxygen, and some food up there. Chairs and boxes were brought up to serve as waiting areas inside the catwalk. Finally, some type of security was needed to prevent people from wandering around on the helipad. Soon, a small squad of staff had the catwalk readied to serve as a holding area while patients waited for the anticipated helicopters.

The Acadian Air Ambulance Service began arriving around three in the afternoon. The commander of the service dropped off a crewmember to help organize the helipad so that no one would get injured on the deck. The crew chief also had a satellite telephone, the most reliable communication available. He could sometimes let us know that a chopper was coming, but occasionally one would arrive unexpectedly. Two might arrive within ten minutes.

Then two hours might elapse until the next chopper showed up. By default, I was in charge of the helipad operations, since it was so crucial to get the intensive care patients out. None of us was experienced in evacuating patients by helicopter, particularly under these conditions. We learned on the run and by trial and error.

The major problem to tackle was physically transporting the patients to the helipad. It took forty-five minutes to transport a patient to the helipad from the time I would first radio the ICU to send a patient up. The drill began when I called to send for a patient to be brought up for chopper evacuation. The nurses then would gather the patient's many tubes, chart, oxygen, and other personal belongings onto the stretcher or into the wheelchair. They would wait for the only functional elevator and go down to the second floor. From there, the entourage would go to the crawlspace connecting the hospital to the parking garage below the helipad. The patient would be passed through the crawlspace on a stretcher to other staff members on the garage side. The staff then loaded the person onto the back of a pickup truck, along with his or her equipment. The truck drove up the ramps to the top of the garage.

The next leg of the trip required carrying the patient and all the equipment up the two sets of metal steps to the roof of the hospital.

After this, the final stretch meant carrying the load of moving flesh and equipment up two more flights of metal steps from the roof to the helipad. The awkwardness and weight of patients on ventilators, or newborns in isolation crates, made it extremely difficult to transport these patients and equipment, such as oxygen tanks, to the helipad.

The other lesson that we quickly learned was that a helicopter was a very precious commodity. If the helicopter happened to land and was not loaded with a patient in a short time, the helicopter would simply take off to fly another mission. Once or twice, a helicopter landed and the patient was still in transit from the hospital, so the chopper crew just left. We quickly developed a system in which patients would be lined up waiting to board helicopters in the covered catwalk. This strategy was risky, since intensive care patients belong in an intensive care unit, not lying exposed to the sun and elements with minimal support. But conditions in the hospital were deteriorating, and generator power was quickly vanishing. By Tuesday night, only minimal electrical power was available. The continued flooding submerged the main generator's electrical switching and caused it to fail. Eric, the physical plant manager, found a small generator, and his electricians used it to power a string of landing lights around our helipad. This innovation allowed us to continue evacuating patients well into the night.

Gradually, all of the intensive care patients and the neonatal intensive care patients left on the choppers. High-risk obstetrical patients left with some of the neonates. Dr. Joe Miller, a perinatologist from LSU, left with one of his high-risk obstetrical patients to fly to Women's Hospital in Baton Rouge, eighty miles away. Most of the ICU patients went to Thibodaux General Hospital, about sixty miles away. Sometimes I had no idea where a particular chopper was going after it left with a patient. All I knew was that wherever it was going had to be better than the worsening conditions at Baptist. Dr. Juan Gershanik, an Argentinean neonatologist, got on a chopper with two preemies, each weighing only about two or three pounds. One of the small infants fit in the palm of his hand, while he manually ventilated the infant through a tube in his airway with his other hand. What a way for these two infants to experience their new world.

By nightfall, we had a rhythm going. The ICU steadily sent patients up to the pad. When the queue in the catwalk shortened, I called on the walkie-talkie for one or two more patients, to be sure we always had patients available to be transported, should the unexpected helicopter stop by. While loading one of the neonatal crates into a chopper, I caught my hand on a sharp metal edge of the helicopter door. The inch-long cut was bleeding, and I found some used gauze to wrap it with. I cleaned it after first aid material arrived two hours later. Even providing first aid for a simple cut was an ordeal for the hospital at this point.

John Walsh walked quickly across the rust-colored helipad toward me after one of the Acadian Air Ambulance helicopters lifted off, his green scrubs and curly black hair blowing in the breeze.

"Hey, John. Welcome to Baptist International Airport," I said. "Will you be traveling first class today, sir?"

"Yes, I will be," John said. "And I'll expect personal attention from the stewardess and prompt service from the on-board bar."

"What's going on? What brings you all the way up here?" I said.

"Look, one of the brothers in the 'hood got stabbed. Somehow they got him to the ER on a boat. The knife wound looks like it's to the abdomen, but I'm worried it might be into the chest, too. He's bleeding all over. We're applying pressure, but we don't have any way of operating on him here. The OR is down. The ER just doesn't have the capability to do what I'd need to do. He's getting fluids and blood. His pressure is okay, but we need to get him someplace where he can get operated on as soon as possible."

"Definitely. We'll put him in the high-priority category. Does he have a chance?"

"Yeah, he could make it to fight again if we can get him operated on fast."

"Okay, go ahead and bring him up. I don't know when the next chopper will be coming or if they can take him, but at least he'll be ready."

"Don't worry. He's already on his way up."

Seconds later, an entourage of nurses, physicians, and staff arrived with a young, muscular man on a stretcher. A tattoo of red thorns ringed the dark skin on his arm. A blood-soaked bandage was wrapped around his upper abdomen and lower chest. Four panting staff members each held a corner of the stretcher, and another was holding up an IV bag.

"You weren't kidding when you said he was on his way up," I said.

"Bring him over here and set him down," John told the worn-out group handling the stretcher.

"Doc, am I going to make it?" the man asked. The crowd of attendants placed him on the ground. His voice was soft, too weak to speak in much more than a whisper. The few words he did say quivered with emotion and betrayed his bravado as a street fighter.

"I hope so. We're going to try to get you on the next chopper if we can," John said.

I could tell the dude knew he was in deep shit. This was not just another trip to the hospital to get sewn up. It was a miracle he even made it to the hospital at all. He could have just died out there in the water.

But I also knew we were in deep shit too. A patient coming in for a stab wound to the belly would usually be a routine process. Labs, X-rays, and transport to the operating room would be as common as turning on the lights. Now, nothing was easy. This patient couldn't get X-rays, since the machines were down. The blood he was receiving was universal blood, since the lab couldn't do a type and cross-match to give him his particular blood type. The building the operating room was in had no electricity. Even transporting patients around the facility was a major ordeal. We were kidding ourselves if we thought we could run a real hospital at this time under these conditions. Our best bet was to serve the people here by getting them out as soon as possible. The longer it went on, the worse it would get.

I talked to the Acadian Air Ambulance commander on the deck and explained the situation to him. He had a reliable satellite radio that he was using to contact the rest of the helicopter squadron. He radioed to his colleagues and told them of the emergency.

"Okay, Doc, I got someone coming, and they'll bring him to the nearest hospital with a functioning OR." He smiled. We both knew that this guy would be dead in twenty-four hours if not for the helicopter commander's intervention.

About thirty minutes later, the street fighter's angel of mercy landed. We quickly loaded him aboard, and within minutes, he flew away into the darkness.

"Where are they going?" I asked the commander.

"They'll start flying toward Baton Rouge and radio the hospitals from the air to see who'll accept him. Lots of hospitals in the surrounding flight paths are filling up fast. Things are changing quickly, and we can't even tell where we're bringing people, because we'll get diverted to another facility along the way that has some capacity. The closer places are almost all packed. We're having to fly all the way to Lafayette now."

"Flying that far takes a long time, and you can't make as many runs."

"Yeah, and our boys are having to even stop to refuel along the way. That really slows things down."

"It must be a madhouse at some of those hospitals, with dozens of patients arriving at their doors all of a sudden."

"It's totally out of control, from what I've heard. They're really trying to help out as much as possible. Once patients are stabilized at that facility, they're trying to arrange ambulance transport to other facilities, so that they can free up their hospital for more evacuees. People are all over the halls in some of those places. But they don't have enough ambulances to transport them out."

"Thanks for all your help with this guy and all the others your company has been rescuing."

"No problem."

John left the helipad and went back down to the hospital. Some of the others in the entourage stayed. Dr. Paul Primeaux, a tall, young anesthesiologist and new on the staff, offered his assistance. He flashed an ear-to-ear smile of his pearly white teeth. His relaxed, tranquil manner portrayed a confidence that everything would be okay. I had seen him around the hospital but had not gotten to know him well. We talked a bit about how the evacuation process worked, so that he could take over if needed.

"Well, how do you think your house did through the storm?" I asked, turning to more personal issues.

"I live on the West Bank. I haven't heard about any levee breaks there, so I hope I'm okay," he said.

"I tried to get to my house last night and again this morning to check on the damage, but debris and water blocked us. My wife and kids left this morning before the water came up again. I'm just hoping they found a way out."

"At least my family wasn't stuck here. They're probably kind of worried about me right now."

"If we can get some boats over here by tomorrow, we should all be fine," I said.

Another chopper approached and drowned out our conversation.

At the evening disaster meeting, the nurses reported that some staff and physicians had left during the small window of opportunity earlier in the morning to get out of the garage. No orthopedists remained in the hospital, and only one surgeon, Dr. John Walsh, had stayed. The physician placed in charge of the oncology unit and bone marrow unit had also abandoned the facility. I appointed another physician to take over that job on the oncology unit and to triage those patients for the next set of evacuations, whenever that would be. One patient had just undergone a bone marrow transplant and was severely immunocompromised. Potent chemotherapy medicines had knocked out his immune system, and he was extremely vulnerable to infections. The only place for that patient to go was to M.D. Anderson, the cancer facility in Houston, which had a bone marrow transplant unit. Administrators worked on transportation for this patient as Susan stood tall and directed the meeting.

Susan next reported that the water level was expected to continue rising throughout the night and might even top the first floor. She said the authorities had decided to go ahead and let the city flood and then repair the breaks in the levees. After the breaks were repaired, they would start pumping the water out. They estimated it might be a month before all the water could be pumped out. The news was all bad.

The realization hit me that New Orleans as I knew it was history. What was going to happen to the city I loved? What about my practice? The patients? The people? The restaurants, the shops? Its quirkiness? It was all gone. An emptiness filled my head as I stared out at the blank wall behind Susan. Thoughts of the meaning of why this happened and what it meant for the future kept clawing at me. My mind had never even formulated any of these questions before, much less tried to answer them.

I left the meeting early, feeling sick and empty inside, and headed back up to the helipad. Steady progress had been made during the past hour. Another five or six people had been airlifted to safety. Paul and I chatted in the moonlight. The confident smile gently stretched across his face, which was stubbled with three days worth of whiskers.

"We sure have a bunch of anesthesiologists in this mess," I said.

"Yeah, it's crazy that we have three of us here and there's not even an operating room for us to work out of. I should be out having a beer."

I liked his sincere, easygoing personality and his spirit of generosity.

"I'll get the first round for us if we ever get out of here," I said.

"Hey, it looks like another one's heading our way," he said as he pointed to a spotlight in the distance.

The chopper steadily approached but then kept on flying to an unknown destination.

"Another false alarm," I said.

"So how did you end up here?" he asked.

"I had this crazy notion that I should help out the community when it needed me. I felt some kind of obligation. A sense that New Orleans was a place where we all helped each other out. Black and white, it didn't matter. It's a unique place. It's been a great community for me and my family. My kids have always thought

I was stupid, but I've always stayed here for hurricanes in the past to fulfill this self-imposed duty to the community. We've never evacuated. In fact, when we're out of town, we actually come back for the storms. That's what we did for Katrina too."

"My wife and I really like it here too. The place just grows on you. It's so horrible to hear about all the looting and crime going on."

Reports and rumors of widespread looting, murders, rapes, and other violence throughout the city had circulated around the hospital since the afternoon.

"I just can't believe the people are tearing up the place like that," I said. "It's so disappointing."

"I just heard that a cop was shot in the face today when he tried to stop a looter."

"You're kidding."

"No. He got sent to West Jeff to get neurosurgery. I think he's doing all right now."

We heard the crackling of gunfire pierce the otherwise quiet darkness off in the distance.

"You heard that?" he asked. "This city is tearing what's left of itself apart."

"What are you going to do when it's all over?"

"I don't see us leaving in spite of all this. If our house is okay and I can get work somewhere now that the hospital's out of commission indefinitely, we'll stay."

"We live in River Ridge," I said. "I think our place is dry. But we have a lot of trees, and I hope none of them fell on the house."

"What are you going to do?" he asked.

"I don't know. We won't be able to practice here for a long time. They're predicting it'll be a month before even all the water gets pumped out. I don't even know where my wife and kids are right now. I'm hoping they're not trapped in the Superdome. I haven't been able to contact them since they left this morning. We'll just have to wait and see what happens."

Helicopters would land sporadically and pick up two or three pregnant women or an intensive care unit patient. We had evacuated about half of the people we had identified as very high risk. The pace was slow and unpredictable, but progress continued.

Sometime after nightfall, Susan made the trek to the helipad. She looked like she was on a mission. Her tall swagger and stern expression commanded my attention.

"Dr. Deichmann, you are sending patients to places that have not formally accepted them," she said. "You just can't do that. We need to contact the receiving facility and get confirmation first." She and her staff had been contacting other hospitals and Tenet headquarters somehow, to make such arrangements. Telephone and cell phone services were still spotty to non-existent, but e-mail and text messaging might have been working.

"Susan, if a helicopter lands and we don't load it up, it's going to take off," I explained. "If that happens, we've just lost the opportunity to get someone out of here. We've already had one helicopter leave empty because we weren't ready fast enough. I'm not letting that happen again."

"The other hospital doesn't even know they are coming."

"Patients are going to die on this catwalk waiting on a confirmation which may not ever come anyway."

"EMTALA requires certain procedures before transferring a patient," she argued. EMTALA is the federal law dealing with hospital transfers.

"Look, some of these chopper pilots aren't even bringing the patients to the hospitals which have accepted them. One of the pilots told me that once in the air, they sometimes are diverted to another facility anyway. These guys are going to fly to the closest hospital and drop off the patients, no matter what you or I say," I responded.

"I don't know. We're not supposed to be doing this."

"We have a lot of patients to evacuate. We need to load patients into the helicopters as fast as possible. Anywhere is safer than this place."

She left in the darkness to make the long walk back into the hospital and tackle a multitude of other problems as the disaster commander. I was thankful that at least I didn't have to deal with the mountain of stress she was carrying. Her usually perfect posture slumped as she stepped away.

We continued to evacuate as fast as the choppers would allow, with little regard to the paperwork. Nothing about what was happening would be via protocol or standard operating procedure. Creative improvisation was the best tool we had if we were to save the two thousand people trapped inside the hospital.

Finally, around eleven at night, the last high-risk person was taken by helicopter from the helipad. The Acadian crew chief gave me the bad news that their service would not be coming on Wednesday. He said that the state and federal officials had taken over the airspace and wouldn't let them fly any longer. The government officials were also taking over the rescue efforts, and would be here in force in the morning to evacuate the whole facility, according to reports he received on his satellite phone.

"Now that those guys are mobilized, they'll have choppers and boats. Y'all be out of here in no time tomorrow," he assured me. "Be sure you have everyone lined up and ready to go so you don't have those long delays in getting people ready for evacuation, like we had earlier today."

"Thanks again for everything," I said. His team had saved the lives of about twenty-five people in the last nine hours. We still had about two thousand more lives inside.

"Don't worry. Y'all gonna be fine," he said and turned away.

He boarded the last helicopter with his buddies and our last ICU patient and took off.

The staff on the helipad was grimy, sweaty, and exhausted after the long day's manual labor under the hot sun. I hadn't had anything to eat since the cup of grits and scrambled eggs earlier in the morning. The merciless heat caused me to make frequent trips to the water bottle, but my hunger now demanded attention. Never had the granola bars waiting for me in my office seemed so appealing.

The helipad became quiet as everyone left. I looked out over the city from the high perch. The surrounding blackness was cut only by the light from random fires burning out of control in the city. The intense silence was striking. No chirping of crickets or humming of cicadae. No owls hooting or bothersome dogs barking. No cars, no music, no voices. The occasional popping of gunfire pierced the shroud of silence. The black shroud of death had a feel too. Death that night felt hot, humid, sweaty, and lonely. The death cloak draped everything I could see or hear as I peered off the edge of the pad. Under its vast stillness, who knew how many thousands of lives had been snuffed out? The city's spirit lay lifeless under its weight too. I felt a strange mix of awe and fright to see death on such a massive, uncaring scale. So this is what death looks, sounds, and feels like?

I said a prayer on the pad to deliver me from its clutches. The chapel was not available.

CHAPTER 4

Wednesday

> *Every living thing that moved on the earth perished—birds, livestock, wild animals, all the creatures that swarm over the earth, and all mankind. Everything on dry land that had the breath of life in its nostrils died. Every living thing on the face of the earth was wiped out; men and animals and the creatures that move along the ground and the birds of the air were wiped from the earth.*

— Genesis 7:21-23

I awoke to a dull thud, thud, thud. My watch said 1:30 AM. My slumber had lasted only an hour. What in the hell was it now? The noise came from the door to the hall and now carried with it the faint sounds of "Dr. Deichmann, Dr. Deichmann." Was I dreaming? I put on some pants and walked in the direction of the exit from the office. The sounds became louder. I opened up another door leading to the exit.

"Dr. Deichmann, are you in there?" someone asked.

"Yeah! I'm in here. Hold on. I'm coming." I hurried to the next door and opened it. One of the security guards, Ms. Ford, stood in the glow of her flashlight.

"We've been trying to get you on the walkie-talkie," she said.

"Well, it doesn't look like it's working anymore," I said.

"Dr. Armington said that some Coast Guard helicopters may be coming. He wants to know if we can reopen the helipad."

"I don't think it's a good idea. Everyone has been up so long. People are tired and need some rest. Besides, it's dangerous to be working up on that thing at night. We already had one person fall off the pad, but he got caught by the fence. Tell him to send them in the morning." *Like we have any control over when they come,* I thought.

"Okay, Doc. I'll let him know. Now I have to get all the way back over there. I didn't know this be a twenty-minute trip. Baby, you gonna wear me out going up and down all these stairs." She turned and headed back toward the dark stairwell.

I went back to sleep as best I could.

At sunrise, I pulled myself off the mat and put on the nasty clothes. *This will be the last time I have to put these stinky things back on,* I thought. *We're getting out of here today.* I filled up the all-important water bottle and ate my last two granola bars. I decided to save the half-full jar of peanut butter, in case I became desperate. I didn't want to rely on the hospital's diminishing stocks of food. Others who had no food needed it more than I did.

I headed over to the ER loading ramp. The water had stopped rising near the top of the street signs. The first floor was spared, and since the ER was located on that level, the loading ramp could still be used for an evacuation route by boat. The boats would have to be the key to the evacuation. Choppers could only take two or three people at a time, and it would be impossible to get two thousand people out without a massive airlift. I knew that if the pace of the evacuation did not pick up today, we could be in for a very long haul. A flotilla of boats was the only sure way of pulling it off.

The stairwell to the fourth floor command center was completely black. The little power from the generator was now gone with the rising water, and no lights were on anywhere. Faint traces of light leaked into the inner hallways by way of the open doors to patient rooms with windows.

The early-morning crisis meeting convened, and Susan announced that we would be rescued by both boats and helicopters that day. She had regained the spring to her step and the smile on her face. I was never sure how she was getting her information. But she said the things I wanted to hear, so I wasn't going to argue. We planned the day's evacuation strategy, and the meeting broke up.

We had learned a lot about efficient evacuation techniques from the day before. Since it took forty-five minutes to get a patient from the hospital to the pad, the key was to have a queue of patients ready to go at the edge of the helipad, inside the catwalk. Backing up the group in the catwalk, a pipeline to the crowds in the hospital needed to be filled with potential evacuees, to replace those in the catwalk who were leaving. Helicopters would land with absolutely no forewarning. No one could predict when this would happen, but we needed to be ready when it did.

The other factor to figure into in the evacuation plan was that some helicopters would take only certain types of people. Some choppers didn't fly to hospitals because of the distance. These crews would only accept healthy people to bring to the airport or some other evacuation staging area close by. Still other choppers might not be able to accommodate stretchers, but could take wheelchair patients. Our plan provided for all these groups to be always at the ready and in the catwalk. One way or another, a helicopter could be packed with appropriate individuals and taken from the facility.

I saw Bill Armington, the mountain-climbing radiologist, after the meeting.

"Hey, what was going on last night up on the helipad?" I asked. "I couldn't believe you were even still awake."

"We had this Coast Guard chopper land out of the blue in the middle of the night," he began. "The crazy thing was the chopper pilot showed up to come get his wife. He jumps out of the chopper with his orange jumpsuit and a helmet the size of a basketball. Then the guy starts running through the hospital with a halogen light, yelling for his wife."

"You've got to be kidding," I said.

"No. He's like an alien from another planet. He's asking everyone if they've seen his wife. Pretty soon, the people lying around in the halls begin to sense his desperation, and everyone starts to panic. He finds the wife, but now the mob starts to chase them as they escape back to the chopper. Hey, they want to be rescued, too. It was wild! A riot almost broke out as they followed him and grabbed at him while he made his way back to the helipad. They both eventually got on the chopper and took off."

"He wasn't going to let his wife be stranded in this pit," I said.

"No way," he said. "He wasn't leaving until he saved her."

"You got some others out, too?"

"Yeah, we got a few Lifecare patients out. Then the choppers stopped coming." Lifecare was a hospital within the hospital. Lifecare Hospital leased the seventh floor of the main building to care for long-term patients. Many of the patients had terminal illnesses, complicated wounds requiring multiple therapies, or long-term use of ventilator machines to breathe.

"It sounds like we'll be getting everyone out today. I'm headed up to the helipad to get things organized up there."

On my journey up to the pad, I stopped to talk to Dr. Skinner. His increasingly ruffled hair only enhanced his professorial look.

"Richard, we've three more deaths," he said in his baritone voice. "They were all no-codes."

A "no-code" patient indicated that the patient did not want to be resuscitated if he stopped breathing or if his heart stopped. The phrase came from the term "code blue," which was announced over the loudspeakers throughout the hospital whenever a patient was found to be in a life-threatening situation. Simultaneously, the beepers and cell phones of the code blue team would go off, sending the team members scurrying to the location of the patient in distress. Doctors, nurses, respiratory therapists, and support personnel would literally run through the corridors to the patient's bedside. The code cart brought by the nurse had all the equipment to shock the heart back to life, begin ventilation through a tube in the airway, and give emergency medications immediately to resuscitate the person. One person compressed the patient's chest, while another would start an intravenous catheter in a vein leading directly to the heart, through which lifesaving drugs would be given. Cardiac monitoring equipment would record the cardiac rhythm throughout the process.

When a person was nearing the end of life and further treatment of his disease was futile, frequently the person would ask not to be resuscitated, in order to avoid prolonging the misery. I was wondering if more patients than usual were declaring themselves to be "no-codes" in view of the misery and futility of all that surrounded them. I also realized that in light of the lack of loudspeakers, beepers, or cell phones, the alarm "code blue" could carry only within earshot. Sick people could be in distress, and there was no efficient way of calling for help. Even if help did arrive, we couldn't provide any kind of serious advanced life support without electricity, running water, or basic sanitary conditions.

I turned my attention back to Dr. Skinner.

"Are they in the chapel too?" I asked.

"Yes. It's getting really hot inside, and I suspect we may notice quite a few deaths if this continues."

"Do you have body bags?" I asked.

"No. All of the body bags are in the basement, under water. The bodies are wrapped in sheets now, and will start to decay fast in this heat."

"Okay. They say we'll be getting out today. Let's see."

I wished him good luck and set out again for the helipad.

When I arrived on the pad, a few people were already wandering around. One woman I recognized from the evening before was a nurse who had helped out, but was another nameless face to me. She was petite and had a head of curly, light-colored hair, and a huge smile.

"Hey, Dr. Deichmann," she said. "I'm Betty Bennett. I'd like to help out today if it's okay."

"Definitely. Look, call me Richard," I said. "The key to keeping this organized is to have a variety of different categories of evacuees available for departure at all times. If they want stretcher patients, we'll have them. If they'll only take ambulatory patients, we'll have them too. Sometimes they only pick up healthy evacuees, so let's have a few of them ready too."

"One thing I noticed yesterday and last night was that security around the perimeter was not too good. It's dangerous to have people walking around all over up here."

"Any suggestions? The air ambulance crew chief also said that was a problem," I said.

"I'm also a captain in the air force, and know how to operate a landing zone. We need to limit access to this area."

"Perfect. I didn't know we had an air force captain to help us. Please direct any staff as you see fit." Finally, we had someone who knew how to really operate a landing zone. If choppers started coming in greater numbers, her expertise could allow much more efficient turnaround time on the pad. Faster turnaround meant greater numbers of people getting out more quickly.

Betty set up a security perimeter around the helicopter landing zone and posted a person at the entrance points to the helipad to limit access. The captain also made sure the pad was clear as helicopters approached. What she couldn't control, though, was the arrival of the helicopters.

By eight AM, we had patients waiting in queues both on the helipad and by the emergency room loading ramp, just as the Acadian chief had recommended. The second floor served as the primary staging area so that no time would be wasted when either the boats or helicopters started arriving. People could be sent for from either evacuation area more easily if they were on the second floor. The water had stopped rising, and the first floor was dry. Our plan was to move those people from the second floor to the first floor if they were evacuating by boats docking at the ER loading ramp. Those leaving by chopper would have access to the parking garage and then the helipad by way of the second-floor crawlspace.

Hour after hour passed, with only an occasional helicopter landing. The government had done a great job of taking control of the airspace and preventing any private helicopters from helping us. But they provided precious little support to replace the loss of the Acadian Air Ambulance service from the night before.

About twenty people languished inside the catwalk, sweating in the unrelenting heat as the sun rose higher. Although we got our sickest patients out the evening before, we still had a number of patients who were quite ill. The ones who were in most urgent need of evacuation were the dialysis patients. Without electricity, these dialysis patients had not been dialyzed for more than four days now. They were getting weaker and more lethargic as the poisons and acids accumulated in their bodies. One was slumped over in his wheelchair, trying to hold on.

To improve the ventilation in the catwalk, we began breaking out the Plexiglas that covered the tunnel. I picked up an oxygen tank and slammed it into the Plexiglas. To my amazement, it bounced right off and almost recoiled out of my hands. I mustered more determination, and with my entire body, I again slammed the green oxygen tank into the thick plastic. A loud explosion boomed, and my left hand felt an immediate electrical pain shooting up my hand into my arm.

My first thought was that the oxygen tank I was holding had exploded. Such an explosion would have meant instant death. Noticing that, in fact, I was still around, I realized that the shattered glass had made all the noise. Blood flowed in a small stream from the back of my left hand, cut by the jagged, broken Plexiglas. I used some of the alcohol which had been brought up to the deck the day before after my first hand injury, and now cleaned the new hand wound. A relatively clean piece of cloth hung from a wheelchair in the catwalk ramp. I used it to wrap around the wound to stop the bleeding and to keep it protected. It also provided symmetry with the bandage already wrapped around my right hand. Sporting makeshift white mittens on both hands, I got to work on the remaining windows.

Eventually, we knocked out just about all of the windows. Wrapping our hands in towels before pounding the oxygen tanks into the windows prevented any further cuts or injuries. The ventilation improved as a slight breeze blew out the hot, stifling air from the tunnel through the new holes. Still, nothing could be done to stop the steady rise in the outside temperature as the day wore on.

Boredom and a general lethargy set in among the whole group of us, as nothing happened hour after hour. Where were the federal and state helicopters that were supposed to be coming? We tried to keep people comfortable by having some more chairs brought up from the hospital. Others just sat on the ground or on boxes. A five-gallon jug of water helped quench people's never-ending thirst in the blazing heat. We rearranged the seating from time to time, to take advantage of minor changes in the light wind, to relieve some of the overwhelming heat. The patients wilted like flowers in a drought.

I got to talking with one of the NOPD officers who was stationed at Baptist. He was a stocky guy with sweat soaking through the blue uniform shirt. A do-rag around his head prevented the sweat from rolling down his forehead into his muddy eyes.

"Man, this is some shit, huh, Doc?" he philosophized.

"You got that right," I agreed.

"The water started coming up at our station and we had to abandon it," he continued. "Everyone's totally scattered now. I can't get in touch with anyone. I have no idea what's happening. The station commander told us just to leave. He said if we wanted to report to our assignments, okay. But he said it's every man for himself. Take care of yourself and your family if you need to. So I came here. I don't know where anyone else is. I don't even know where my people are."

"How'd you end up taking on this job, anyway?" I asked. "Look at all the mess you're in now."

"Doc, I came over to NOPD from another police department in a different city a couple of years ago. The pay was a little better. I wanted to do something different too. But I never expected to see some of the shit I've seen in this job. This is a rough place. People are crazy out there. And now this."

"So what are you going to do after you get out of here?"

"I have no idea. All I know is things is gonna get really bad out there, the longer this goes on. Doc, things is gonna get bad here too. I gotta tell you. You got a bad situation on your hands here. Your Guard dudes have all gone, and there's only two of us from NOPD here now."

"I didn't know the National Guard had left. What happened to them?"

"They all got sent over to the Superdome."

"How'd they get there?" I asked.

"Probably by boat," he said.

"How long are you going to stay?"

"I don't know. I might need to take care of my people. But I don't know where they are. I think my house is totally gone, 'cause I lived in New Orleans East." He sipped on his water bottle and turned to stare at the vast expanse of water from the helipad. "And, Doc, once I do get out of here, I don't think I wanna come back either."

A random military helicopter would land every two hours or so and take two or three patients. The day was wearing on, and not much progress was being made. Our spirits waned under the oppressive sun.

Nearing midday, a commotion suddenly broke out on the other side of the helipad. One of the civilian sentries on the helipad was trying to prevent three people from walking across the helipad. I walked over to see what was going on.

"Doc, these people don't belong here," the nervous, inexperienced sentry said. He pointed to three skinny folks with wet, dirty clothes. "They came up from the water and just walked all the way up here. They don't have wristbands either."

They started shouting at once.

"We want to be rescued!" demanded the one with the cornrows and flip-flops. Her shirt had lost two buttons.

"Nowhere for us to go," her teenage companion added. He deferred to her as he stroked the stubble on his chin.

"We ain't leaving," the third one shouted in my face. "I don't care what nobody says. Nobody's kicking me outta here!" The apparent ringleader made the announcement with a mouth and lips proportionately oversized for her thin face. Her sharp, haggard features gave the words even more impact.

The sentry and I looked at them. Weren't they some of the looters we had noticed last night cruising in the flat-bottom boat in the street next to the hospital with TVs aboard? I couldn't be sure. But I didn't have the heart to send them back out into the water.

"Okay. Okay. Settle down," I said. "We'll let you stay. But y'all aren't going to be the first to go. We have a lot of sick people to get out. Y'all won't be leaving until we get the sick patients out first. Now I don't want any trouble from y'all. Is that clear?"

"We not gonna be no trouble," the ringleader said. "We just wanna get outta here."

"The first sign of trouble from any of you and I'm sending you out. You hear?"

They nodded.

I walked them to the back of the evacuation line in the catwalk tunnel and found a seat for one of them. The other two sat on the floor, leaning against the wall. I gave them some water and went back to the area near the helipad. The NOPD officer was back there and promised to keep an eye on them.

During some of the down time, I went back downstairs to check on what was happening in the hospital. Captain Betty took over on the helipad while I was gone. I caught up with John in the ER. His green scrubs were soaked with sweat.

"We have everybody lined up and ready to go from the ER loading ramp, but no boats are coming," John said. "We heard we might be getting some state police boats here this afternoon. It's so hot in here!"

We walked out to the ramp, where dozens of people waited at the waterline. We leaned on a brick wall and looked out at the water.

Tree limbs, plastic jugs, driftwood, and Styrofoam littered the murky water. Gasoline had leaked from the many submerged cars around the hospital. The water had large pools of petroleum products floating about and lapping against the hospital walls. The eerie magenta, purple, and emerald sheen of gasoline surrounded us in a toxic stew. I suddenly was worried that if the water caught on fire, the hospital would burn down faster than a tinder box. Hadn't the Cuyahoga River in Cleveland caught fire decades before from oil pollution? We had no running water and no sprinkler system. People would be trapped in the inferno, their only possible escape being the flaming water around the building. I shuddered at the thought.

"John, suppose this place catches on fire?" I asked.

"Hopefully, people have enough sense not to toss a lit cigarette into the water," he said. "That's about the only way it could possibly get any hotter inside."

"You're right about that. We knocked out a bunch of windows up by where we are and it helped some. Let's knock out some windows to improve ventilation here in the hospital. I think it would help."

I asked René about busting out the windows before we started further damaging his facility. He agreed to the proposal as he wiped the beads of sweat off his forehead. Soon, a team put together by Dave Goodson and Eric Yancovich were breaking out windows all over. They took the precaution of wrapping their hands with towels to prevent any hand injuries from the razor-sharp glass. John didn't have the resources to be treating any really serious lacerations that might occur should an artery get nicked. The crash of shattering glass followed by the splash of the pieces hitting the water below broke the cone of silence around us. As much as it was a remedy for the heat, it was also a way of asserting our aliveness as the silence tried to snuff us out.

John and I went to fill our water bottles with the lifesaving liquid.

"I think my house is flooded. It's only about ten blocks away," he said. There was not much to joke about lately.

"I'm sorry to hear that, John. I hope it's not too bad. How about your family?"

"They're up in Alexandria. They're okay."

"I'm not sure where Cecile and the kids are," I said. "They left yesterday morning during that small window when the water had gone down. I haven't heard from them since. I'm worried that they got stuck or may have ended up in the Superdome. Suppose they're in the Convention Center?" I looked away, staring off across the water as my voice trailed off.

"Don't worry. They're probably all right," he said, looking in the other direction too.

I unexpectedly lost any interest in talking, and needed a little time to myself.

"I'm going to head back up," I said. "Let me know if boats start to come. We aren't getting any activity up top. I'll start sending people back downstairs to you if you start to get a lot of activity."

"All right. Take care. I'll come get you if we start to get a lot of boats."

I took my time getting back upstairs, avoiding people along the way as much as possible.

Around noon, an NBC reporter walked up to the helipad from the first floor with his cameraman. This evidence of the outside world startled me. I wondered how he had found us. If he could get to the hospital, why couldn't government officials also get here and get us out? The isolation was unbearable. The government had stopped private helicopter services from assisting us, and now left us even more stranded. The negligence was mind-boggling.

"Hey, Doc, you in charge up here?" he asked.

"Yeah," I said. "What are you doing up here?"

"We've been going around by boat—reporting on the flooding, looting, crime, everything. It's unbelievable. It's just surreal."

"What's going on out there?" I was starved for information.

"We passed dead bodies floating in the water on the way over here. There's massive flooding as far as I could see. Looting is going on all over, particularly downtown. The Superdome has thousands of people stuck there, fighting for food and water. Massive destruction all over, with houses collapsed, trees down, fires. It's the worst situation I've ever reported on. It's so sad, it's really affecting me being here, and I don't even live here. I just don't know how this place is going to ever recover from this."

A heaviness came over me again. It was the only firsthand account I'd received of what was going on since the flood started. I didn't have access to radio or TV, and rumors were the only news available. My thoughts again turned to Cecile and my daughters. Were they safe? Did they get out, or had they been trapped by the rapidly rising water? Were they among the mobs in the Superdome? What about my beloved city? "How is this place going to recover from this?" the reporter had asked me.

Katrina was exposing a part of this community that I'd not experienced. Was it my naiveté? How could the citizens turn against each other so quickly? How could the city, state, and federal officials abandon us at the hospital as one by one, more people died? Where were the many boats that in the past fishermen and neighbors would bring in to save those stranded on rooftops? We needed boats that could evacuate five or ten at a time. We were never going to get out of here with helicopters taking two or three at a time. How could the community betray us like this?

"Can you get a message out for us?" I asked him. "We need some help in the worst kind of way."

"Sure, we'll set up for a short interview," he said.

I composed myself and gathered my thoughts for the interview. I wanted to be brief and stay on point.

"We have Dr. Richard Deichmann, the chief of the medicine department here at Memorial Medical Center," the reporter began. "Doctor, tell us what the conditions are like here in the hospital." The camera was rolling in the glaring sunlight on top of the helipad.

"The facility lost its electrical power on Sunday night and now has lost its generator power," I said. "It's very hot inside and there's little ventilation. We are running short on food and water. We are also running low on oxygen. There's no running water."

"How many people are inside?"

"We have about two thousand people total. We have about two hundred patients left to be evacuated. We got about twenty-five of our very sickest patients out last night. Neonates, pregnant women, and ICU patients. We're in urgent need of boats to come rescue the large number of people who remain here. The situation is very serious, and we have people who were healthy becoming patients, due to the heat and stress. Those who were already sick are rapidly getting worse and need evacuation immediately. We still haven't gotten out all of our dialysis patients. They'll die without dialysis soon. Please send us help as soon as possible."

The interview was over. Would anyone even hear it? Would anyone bother to respond?

The reporter and cameraman left the helipad and entered the hot catwalk tunnel on their way back downstairs. The woman with the big mouth and haggard face sprang up from her seat toward the back and ran toward the reporter, with her two friends right behind her. A middle-aged man in a plain white T-shirt looked on with eyes wide open.

"We're dying in here," she screamed, grabbing at the reporter. "Get us out of here. Help us. Help!"

"Tell people we're dying," the one with the flip-flops yelled into the camera. "Hey, out there, come get us!"

"We need help, man. Where is everybody? Come here, now." The man with the facial stubble also joined the fray.

The cameraman quickly covered the camera to protect it as the group pushed and grabbed at him too. The reporter backed away as the NOPD officer with the bandanna quickly separated the group.

"Hey, I told y'all to settle down and not cause any trouble!" I yelled. These hoods were getting everyone in the tunnel anxious with the outburst.

"We gonna die! We gotta get outta here," the ringleader screamed.

"That does it. Y'all are out of here." I turned to the NOPD cop. "Officer, get these people out of this facility. They don't belong here and are trespassing and stirring up trouble. Get them out of here."

"You not gonna put us out in the water, huh?" the ringleader asked.

"I don't know where you're going to go. I just know you're not going to be in this hospital. Now get out of here."

"I'll take care of them," the officer said as he and another man led them off.

The reporter and cameraman rearranged their clothes and each looked to be sure that the other was okay.

"Doc, we need to leave. Good luck." They hurried out of the back of the tunnel to go down to the boat awaiting them far below. Would the outside world get their message?

Betty, Paul, and I went among the people languishing in the tunnel, to give them water and arrange for them to get some food. About thirty minutes after a runner went for food, he came back with a small box of ham sandwiches. We passed them out, along with a few cookies. I ate my sandwich and nibbled on a piece of dry sausage, washing it down with gulps of water.

I went back down to the hospital to find a restroom. The men's room smelled like an unventilated Port-a-Potty in summer. The ceramic tile room was dark except for the meager light from my flashlight. The unflushed stool and urine in the toilets seemed particularly noxious in the supposedly sterile confines of a hospital. I made my contribution and left.

"Doctor Deichmann, can I talk with you?" Susan stopped me in a quiet hallway while I was returning upstairs.

"Sure. What's going on?" I asked.

"This is a really awful subject. I don't even know how to bring it up."

"We're definitely dealing with a lot of awful things around here. What is it?"

"Well, if things keep getting worse around here, what are we going to do with all the do-not-resuscitate patients? Would euthanasia be the humane thing to do?"

The question startled me. "Things are bad here, but they're not that bad," I said. "The DNRs are low priority on the list, but we still plan to evacuate them. Besides, euthanasia's illegal. If a patient seems to be in a lot of pain, we can give them medication just like we normally would. There's not any need to euthanize anyone. I don't think we should be doing anything like that."

Susan's eyes were moist in the indirect light from the windows two rooms away. She had been under a tremendous strain as the disaster commander. Now she was addressing this unthinkable issue. She seemed relieved with my response.

"Susan, you're doing a good job under these conditions," I said.

"Thanks," she said without much conviction. She turned and walked alone down the dim hallway. Her posture again had just the slightest slump to it.

Shortly after I arrived back to the pad, a large, lumbering airplane approached the skies over the hospital. It seemed to be suspended in midair, it was moving so slowly.

"Hey, that's *Air Force One*," Paul said, his half-smile directed to the sky.

"A lot of good he's doing for us up there," I said. The vast difference in the conditions the president was enjoying and the misery we were experiencing at the moment was on stark display. What was he thinking as he surveyed his kingdom of infidels who had voted against him in the last election? Was it a media-driven fly-over to show some façade of concern? Where was the assistance of the federal government with its vast resources? He had promised all the assistance the government could provide before the storm had struck. Homeland Security had received billions of dollars of funding to protect us, the people. This is what the citizens received for that purchase.

"You know, he doesn't have a clue about what's going on down here," Paul said.

"Yeah. If our National Guard guys were here instead of getting shot at in Iraq, we would've been out of here by now," I said. "Our own guys from Louisiana would know exactly what to do. They would've been around here with hundreds of boats, and have maintained order. This is crazy, trying to rescue all the people in the city by helicopter."

Air Force One slowly lumbered toward the east. I turned away and headed to the relative shade of the catwalk.

Over the next two hours, two more random Coast Guard choppers came and went. We were able to at least finish the evacuation of most of the dialysis patients, with the total of about five choppers that had landed so far that day. The last two remaining dialysis patients sat drooped in their wheelchairs, waiting for a chopper to bring them to a dialysis unit.

The last helicopter had dropped off a special communications radio, and showed Betty how to use it. He also told her of the frequency to the Central Disaster Command Center that had been set up by the authorities in the city.

Betty dialed in the frequency.

"This is Captain Bennett, U.S. Air Force, over."

No reply.

"Repeat, this is Captain Bennett, U.S. Air Force, calling from Baptist Hospital, over."

"Captain Bennett, this is Central Command, do you read?" the radio crackled back.

Betty and I grinned at each other. At last we had contact with the outside world.

"Yes," Betty responded. "We are in urgent need of evacuation. We have over two thousand people here, including two hundred patients. Our generator is out. We have about seven or eight dead."

"We can't come for you now. The priority is still to pick people out of the water and off rooftops. Is there any assistance we can provide until we can get there?"

Betty and I looked at each other and blurted out things we could use to each other.

"Oxygen, a generator, body bags," I said.

"Satellite telephone, walkie-talkie, and chargers," she continued.

"Batteries and flashlights."

"How many body bags?"

"We don't have any. Ask for twenty," I said.

"We better ask for fifty. That'll give them a better idea of how serious it is," Betty said.

"Okay."

She got back on the radio seconds later. "Central Command, this is Captain Bennett. We need oxygen, a generator with fuel, flashlights, batteries, satellite phones and walkie-talkies with chargers, and fifty body bags."

"Roger. We'll see what we can do. We'll need to keep the airtime down. We have a lot of traffic on this frequency."

"I'll call on the hour and keep the radio off until then to conserve batteries."

"Okay. Talk to you at two. Out."

Betty clicked off the radio.

"You know what, Betty?" I said. "Even if we get the walkie-talkies and chargers, we don't have any sockets to plug them into."

"Oh, well. We'll worry about that when and if they come."

About a half hour later, a Coast Guard helicopter flew by in a semi-circle and approached for a landing.

Betty and I smiled at each other. Maybe our luck was finally changing.

"It looks like the Central Command is sending us our first shipment," Betty said to me.

"Yeah, and we can load it up with some more people for shipment out, too," I said. "They responded pretty fast to our call."

The orange-and-white helicopter landed, and a serviceman jumped out. I went over to help him unload, with the roar of the motor drowning out any other sound.

The serviceman put a headset on me so we could talk. Six people stared shell-shocked out from the cargo hold at me. Their clothes were torn and ragged, their skin sunburned, their blank faces emotionless. They had seen death up close and personal.

"Sir, I have six people we picked off roofs that I would like to drop off here," the serviceman said.

I looked at the faces of the evacuees. They had been stranded on rooftops or in the blazing heat of attics since Monday. Almost certainly they had witnessed friends or family drowning or dying from exposure.

"We're trying to evacuate this facility," I said. "We don't have any electricity. Our food and water are low. We have two thousand people we need to get out. I'm sorry. We just can't accept any more people." I felt so guilty not being able to help.

"Doc, please. We need to drop these off ASAP to fly more of these rescue missions. There are hundreds more out there."

"Look, I tell you what I'll do. If you take my last two dialysis patients to a hospital so they can get dialyzed, I'll trade you for the six people in the cargo hold."

"Where do they need to go?"

"Either Thibodaux or Baton Rouge. They'll die if they don't get dialyzed soon."

"That's a long way. I'll have to check." He switched frequencies on his headset radio and talked to the pilot.

"No deal, Doc," he said after conferring with the pilot. "We're gonna take off and find someplace else for the folks in the cargo hold. But we're gonna try to get someone else to come for your dialysis patients. Good luck."

"I wish we could help," I said. "Thanks for all your work out there."

I went back and told Betty what happened. Our luck was not changing after all.

For the rest of the afternoon, Betty faithfully checked in hourly on the radio. As the hours wore on, she would tune in to get any new information. A helicopter dropped off an oxygen tank in the late afternoon. We both laughed when a crew left us two boxes of antibiotics used to treat vaginal infections, and a couple of boxes of Vienna sausages. No batteries, generator, or flashlights. The body bags never would arrive. My eyes widened when Betty noticed a new satellite phone in the shipment. I took it from its box, read the directions, and turned on the power. Hope faded when I dialed a number and got the generic female electronic voice telling me that the service I was trying to use had not been subscribed to.

After waiting around some more, I decided to stroll down to the ER to get any new information that might have trickled in. Paul and Betty would handle loading people onto any choppers that might show up.

I wanted to check out the situation on some of the hospital floors on the way down. Most of the hospital rooms were empty now. Patients had been moved to staging areas on the first and second floors. There was an eeriness about the dark, empty corridors. Old water bottles, discarded clothes, old food, and trash littered the floors. Many of the toilets had been used and, unflushed, produced a foul sewage smell. The fetid smells were aggravated by the heat. No breeze was blowing, and these inside parts of the facility felt like a steam room. An occasional straggler would walk by, possibly trying to recover something he had forgotten or trying to scavenge a spare water bottle. The conditions were far too uncomfortable for patients. Even healthy evacuees avoided strolling around in the dark, spooky Turkish bath inside.

The previous strategy of physicians staffing a particular nursing unit no longer had any purpose, since there weren't any patients and hardly any staff in any of the nursing units. The staff and physicians followed the patients to wherever they had moved for staging. The sicker patients were given higher priority and moved to a staging area closer to the actual evacuation site. Patients had gotten all jumbled together and were no longer identifiable by which nursing unit they had been on. Anticipating imminent evacuation, everyone was tending to congregate near these staging areas. Since hardly any evacuation was occurring, hundreds of people accumulated in these areas.

The second floor was a sea of humanity. Dozens of windows had been broken out either intentionally or by the storm, and provided the slightest hint of ventilation. The smell of sweat and the moans, coughs, and common chatter resembled an overcrowded refugee camp in a war zone. A foodservice line rationed out prepackaged snack foods, cookies, crackers, and pieces of fruit. René passed out food and tried to keep spirits up with his Cajun twang. Sean, his stocky arms glistening with sweat, offered soft drinks or water to the thirsty mob. An armed guard sat next to the Abita water dispenser.

A wiry woman in her thirties came running up to me in a lobby near the street. Her face was strained and her mascara was running.

"Doctor, what are you doing about the sex offenders?" she demanded. Her voice had the urgent firmness of someone expert at lodging effective complaints.

"The sex offenders?" *What in the hell is she talking about?* I wondered.

"Yes. Sex offenders. You don't even know if you have any sex offenders here. We need to identify the sex offenders and separate them from the rest of us."

"I haven't heard about any problems with sex offenders here."

"Well, I think there are some here. We have all these children running around. It's a very dangerous situation. What are you going to do about it, Doctor?"

"Do you know of any sex offenders in the hospital?"

"No."

"Have you seen anybody that looks suspicious?"

"I'm not sure. They don't go around with a sign saying 'I'm a sex offender,' you know," she said.

"We just don't have any way of identifying them and separating them," I said. "I don't think it's a big problem for us now. But if you see or hear of any inappropriate sexual activity, let me know."

"You might not think of it as a problem, but they shouldn't be evacuating to the hospital in the first place."

"Look, I'm focused on trying to get you and everyone else out of here as soon as possible. The sooner you're out of here, the sooner you'll be safe from sex offenders and all the other risks you face here. Let me go to check on the boats downstairs. Get with me if anything suspicious happens."

While she was talking, I could hear the unmistakable loud engine noise of an airboat from the water below. I didn't feel like debating about potential perverts when it looked like some boats were finally arriving.

I took the steps to the first floor, where hundreds more were mulling about. Before I could get down to the ER loading ramp to see John, a group of three people came up to me. One of them was a staff member, and they were worked up about something.

"What are we going to do with our pets?" one of the women asked. Her green shirt and white shorts were ringed with dark, random lines of dirt.

"Well, I know they won't let you take pets on the helicopters," I said.

"Yeah, I know," she said. "But they're not letting me take my dog on the boat either. I'm not leaving my dog behind."

"Well, that's your choice."

"They can't just make us leave our dog behind to die. I'm not going to do it."

"We're in a really awful situation here. Believe me. I know. It's going to be a hard choice."

"He's just going to starve or die of thirst."

A staff member in a yellow pastel shirt overhearing the exchange hugged her and tried to console her. Her concerned eyes offered the lady a sense of caring.

"We are going to evacuate out everyone we can," I said. "If you want to wait until the end to make up your mind, that's okay. But if I were you, and I was offered a ride out of here, I wouldn't pass it up. There might not be the chance to get both you and your dog out of here later, but you could wait and see."

"You can say anything you want, but I'm not leaving." She and her friend turned and walked away.

"Lots of people are worried about their pets," the staff person said. "There are boats outside now, but some people are refusing to get on without their pets."

Images of losing Maggie just three days before kept bouncing up to my consciousness. I knew what that felt like. But I still couldn't understand putting one's own life in jeopardy by refusing a rescue because of a pet. Did people realize how serious the situation here was?

"I think that people will have to end up leaving a lot of these pets here," I responded.

"Isn't there anything we can do?"

"We can't make anyone leave. But if they want to wait until everyone is evacuated and then re-assess the situation, they can."

"What are we going to do with all the animals left behind?" the staff woman persisted. "What's going to happen to them?"

I was losing my patience.

"I don't know what's going to happen to them," I said. "I do know that I'm not going to do anything about them because I'm too worried about trying to get the humans out of here, not the animals." My frustration continued to bubble over. "Anyone who wants to stay in here after everyone else has evacuated can stay and see what it's like being in here all by themselves. Wondering if someone is going to come for them and their animals. Searching for water for themselves. Wondering how they are going to get food for themselves. If they do that, they might be faced with a really bad decision, one they'd really regret. Whether or not to eat their pets to avoid starvation."

Was this still really me saying this kind of stuff?

The staff member stared at me. Her usually rosy cheeks had lost their color. She was speechless at the horror of what I had suggested. She left without even saying good-bye. I later found out she had a dog that she, too, was trying to evacuate with.

I weaved my way through the hundreds of sweaty bodies to the ER loading ramp. I saw John near a broken brick wall bordering the water-filled street. The bottom of his grungy green scrub pants were wet to the mid-calf. The sounds of the airboats drowned out normal conversation.

"John, what happened to the wall?" I shouted.

"We got a sledge hammer and knocked it out so the boats could come right up here and use this as a dock," he yelled back.

People boarded the airboats by stepping from the edge of the elevated loading ramp through the break in the wall and down to the boat below. The water level was about two feet below the edge of that part of the concrete ramp. Two people helped each person board the boat, and another helped them get seated once on board. The older evacuees needed lots of help to prevent them falling into the water. Some of the lighter ones were just lifted up and placed onto the boat.

"Some organization having to do with hunting and fishing showed up about a half hour ago with this fleet of airboats," John continued. "The problem is they can't take anyone who can't walk, and each boat can only hold about three or four people. I think the state police came with a boat, too."

"At least something's happening."

"It's helping people's spirits to see that finally a steady evacuation is going on."

"Where are they bringing the people?"

"I think they're bringing them over to the corner of St. Charles and Napoleon. I'm not sure what's happening after that. They might be shuttling them to the Convention Center or to the airport from there. Anyplace is better than here," he said.

"You got that right. How many boats do they have anyway?"

"I'm not sure, around four or five. There's a really big one that came by they use for those swamp tours over on the West Bank. That sucker loaded up about thirty people. We really need more of those."

"Man, that's really great news. How long are they going to stay?"

"They said they are going to get everyone out by tonight."

"Thank you, Jesus. We're getting out of here!" I was smiling from ear to ear. This concerted effort really could move everyone out if the boats kept running and were joined by others.

I helped load a few people onto the boats. Then I walked over to assist with crowd control. People tried breaking in line to be sure they didn't miss out on being rescued.

The loud boats landed, took on three or four passengers, and quickly took off. Another would be waiting to dock right behind. The process was the most regular attempt at a real evacuation we had seen so far. If another big swamp tour boat showed up, the hospital would be empty tonight. I was giddy with excitement.

"John, I'm going back to the helipad and start sending people down, since not too much is happening up there."

"Wait awhile before you go to all that effort. We've got so many already down here, I don't know what we'd do with a bunch more."

"Okay. Keep up the good work," I said as I left.

The effort of going up and down to the helipad in the overwhelming heat steadily sapped my energy. I felt as if my body was enduring a twenty-four-hour jungle endurance race. The heat was inescapable. My pace slowed as fatigue and soreness set in. Now it took me twice as long to make the trip up to the pad.

Good news awaited me on top.

"We had a couple of choppers come while you were goofing off," Paul said. His big smile confirmed that he must have some particularly positive development.

"Excellent," I said.

"The last two dialysis patients are gone now."

"I'm so glad they're out of here. They couldn't have made it much longer."

"Yeah, the heat was really getting to them and the last two were really lethargic. The last one left around three thirty."

"I have good news for you, too," I said. "There's an armada of airboats shipping people from the loading ramp at the ER. They're making some serious progress. If they get some more boats, we could be out by tonight."

"Should we start sending people down there from here?" he asked.

"No. Let's hold off until they clear out some of the people down there first. Besides, they can't take most of these people because they're too sick. They're only taking ambulatory people right now."

The people in the catwalk tunnel sat quietly on boxes and chairs, sweating and clinging to their water bottles. The frustration and fear showed on their faces as they gazed off into the distance. The heat stifled conversation. The effort just wasn't worth it. I took up a place next to a black man in his fifties and sweated in silence with him. Random people would walk up to the top to see what was going on and leave.

Greg Vorhoff walked across the pad toward me. Greg was a cardiologist whom I had worked with for twenty years. He was thoughtful, dedicated, and had a deep-rooted sense of duty. He loved to talk, and sometimes just wouldn't shut up. As he talked, hand gestures helped mold and emphasize his words in proportion to his passion at the time. In our conversations during the crisis so far, he was appalled that we could be suffering under such conditions with no one coming to help us. His determined stroll meant that he was up to something.

"Richard, I don't think people on the outside realize how serious our situation is. If they did, there would be a massive rescue effort going on here now," he said. His hands quickly sculpted each phrase as he talked.

"Greg, you're probably right. But what can we do about it?"

"I'm going to get some help."

"How are you going to do that?"

"I'm going to get on one of these airboats and personally find the authorities and get them to send more boats here."

"Where are you going to go?" I asked.

"I don't know. But I'll find TV reporters, Nagin, the police chief, whoever I need to. We need help. People are dying down there," he said, pointing to the hospital below.

"It might be dangerous."

"I don't care. I'm getting some help for you, Richard."

"Good luck, Greg."

Greg left. I would not see him again for the duration of the ordeal.

After getting on an airboat, he told me weeks later, he traveled to the corner of St. Charles and Napoleon avenues. He slogged through the water to the dry neutral ground on St. Charles Avenue. Dressed only in his green scrubs, he began walking toward the airport, about twenty miles away. The street was completely depopulated. After walking about three miles, he finally saw another person. The man approached Greg wearing only some tattered clothes.

"Give me all your money," he said. Greg suspected the man was about to pull a gun on him.

"You've got to be kidding, man. I don't have any food, water, or money. Besides, what could you spend it on now?" Greg said. "I'm trying to find some help." He turned his pockets inside out as proof.

"Oh." The dude nonchalantly turned away and kept on walking.

Greg made the turn up Carrollton Avenue and walked another mile or so until he was almost back in the flooded part of town again. He had now walked five or six miles. A pickup truck drove slowly around the downed oak trees, power lines, and debris. It was the first motorized vehicle he had seen since getting off the boat. The driver pulled up to the left of him and opened the passenger door.

"Hey, what are you doing walking around here?" he demanded.

Greg turned, this time definitely finding a gun pointed at him. "What is this?" Greg said. "You're the second guy to hold me up in the last thirty minutes. I'm just trying to get some help for everyone who's trapped at Baptist Hospital. And I don't have any money."

"I'm not trying to rob you. You just can't be too careful around here right now. Here, get in. I'll drive you to a staging area I know about."

Greg got in and they drove upriver along River Road. The air-conditioned pickup drove past Ochsner and on to Causeway Boulevard. After turning onto Airline Drive, they eventually reached the Sam's Club parking lot. Emergency vehicles with their engines off filled the large blacktop lot. Greg got out of the truck to find someone in authority. The unknown pickup truck driver slipped away.

Greg recognized Harry Lee standing between some police cruisers. Lee was the rotund sheriff of Jefferson Parish, and had more political power than the rest of the parish's politicians put together.

"Sheriff Lee, I'm Dr. Greg Vorhoff. I just hitched a ride over here to get help for the two thousand people trapped in Baptist Hospital," he said. I could imagine his hand gestures getting fired up.

"The buses. I can't get the buses," Lee said. His full, red face was sweating profusely. His uniform was soaked. His jowls jiggled from side to side as he shook his head while he talked.

"People are dying in that hospital right now," Greg pressed on. "We've got to get them out. Now."

"They won't give me the buses. I need the buses. Where are they?"

"Sheriff, we need to send boats over to get them out. Can you do that?"

"The buses. Get me the damned buses." The sheriff was incapacitated with the frustration over the lack of buses.

Greg was getting nowhere with his pleadings, so he walked around to find someone else who might help. He saw Eddie Compass, the chief of police for the New Orleans Police Department, sitting in a chair by himself. His face was slumped down into his hands.

"Chief Compass, I'm Dr. Vorhoff from Baptist Hospital. I just got here to try to get some help. We have about two thousand people trapped there. Some are dying. They need to be rescued today."

Compass lifted his heavy head. His eyelids drooped and sweat ran down from his close-cropped hair. He stared blankly at Greg for a few seconds. Without saying anything, he shook his head from side to side and slowly lowered his face back down to his hands.

"Chief, are you going to do anything?" Greg asked again.

The man was unable to respond. He had seen the complete disintegration of law and order in the city that he had sworn to protect. At least one of his officers had already committed suicide from the stress. Scores of police had deserted. Still others had become looters themselves. Many other police officers stayed on the job, but there was no command or control, given the lack of communications.

Greg heard of the evacuation staging area developing at the cloverleaf of I-10 and Causeway Boulevard. He figured maybe someone there might be able to do something. He caught a ride from Sam's Club to the major intersection, about five miles away. Thousands of evacuees were being dropped off there in the grassy fields by helicopters and emergency vehicles. He tried to redirect some of the buses to the area around St. Charles and Napoleon, without any success. He stayed around assisting with some of the sicker evacuees and triaging them onto buses for transport to Baton Rouge.

He eventually ended up in Baton Rouge that night. The next day, he began helping out at the Pete Maravich Assembly Center on the LSU campus, and informing every official he could find of the unfolding disaster at Baptist. The Assembly Center housed hundreds of evacuees from New Orleans, many of whom were in need of medical care. Greg worked at the Center for a second day. But when a security guard pulled a gun on him and accused him of stealing a doughnut, Greg decided he had served enough. He had grown tired of people pointing guns at him. He got in touch with his family and got out of Baton Rouge to join them.

Now, up on the helipad, Captain Betty and I wondered about the success of Greg's scouting trip. Reports from downstairs indicated the boats were still running, but no additional boats had come. The capacity of the current fleet couldn't come close to evacuating the facility today. We had no success in convincing the Central Command to commence an urgent evacuation of our site either. We couldn't even get them to drop off the body bags. Our spirits began to sink once again.

"Hey, what's that guy doing?" I asked, looking over toward a thin, balding man. He was running around the helipad with a massive banner. A woman serving as his assistant held up the other end.

"I don't know, but he's not supposed to be running around up there," Betty said, looking out toward the helipad.

"Help, we're dying! Someone, somewhere, help us," he yelled to the sky. Two hospital sheets joined together served as the banner. It read "HELP! WE'RE TRAPPED AND DYING!"

It was the same person who had been wandering around on the helipad when the news reporter had been up here. He was the pale, middle-aged guy with the white T-shirt and the bulging eyes. One of the staff members had mentioned to me earlier that someone matching his description was running wild around the hospital corridors with a banner and yelling that we were all going to die.

"Save us. Help!" He kept running around, yelling to the sky.

"What are you doing?" I asked as I approached him.

"I'm calling for help. No one else is doing anything."

"We're trying to get people out as fast as possible."

"No one knows how bad things are for us. If they did, they would've come to rescue us by now. I'm getting the word out."

"We have some boats loading people up down by the ER," I reassured him.

"No. They stopped," he said.

Now my eyes widened. Why did they stop? What had happened?

"Well, stop running around yelling and waving this thing around," I told him. "No one can hear you and it's not doing any good."

"I'm not going to stop. We need to let the outside world know we need help."

"Look, all you're doing is getting the people around here upset. We need to try to stay calm."

"Who's getting upset?" he screamed.

"I am. So give me the damned banner right now." I grabbed the banner out of his hands and wadded it up. "Now get out of here and stop stirring people up."

He and his helper sulked away. Panic was spreading like an out-of-control growth of kudzu on a hot summer hillside. I began to fear that a mob from within the hospital might take things in their own hands. The situation could easily turn into a scene from *Lord of the Flies* and a contest of survival of the fittest.

I needed to go back down to find out why the airboats stopped running.

"John, what the hell happened?" I asked.

"They said they had to stop at five," he said. "The state police and the volunteers with the airboats got about five hundred people out. Then they just pulled out."

"Shit. What are you talking about? That means we still have about fifteen hundred people to evacuate."

"They said they're too worried about security. The state police said no more helicopters are coming either because of the security situation."

"If it's too dangerous for the state police, where does that leave us?" I asked in exasperation.

"They said they'd be back tomorrow. Most all the people they took could walk. So we still have the sicker ones here."

"But we have lots of light left, and there's no reason we couldn't keep going at least until dark."

"You can't argue with those guys. They won't listen. You know the biggest problem? These state troopers and National Guard guys are all from out of town. They don't know the culture down here. They hear about some black dudes shooting and looting, and they freak. Then the out-of-town cops see all these blacks in the hospital and in the neighborhoods around here. It gets the cops worried one of them is going to start shooting. They freak all over again. But they don't realize that the vast majority of the brothers are as scared as we are and are just trying to escape this shit."

"I hear you. They really ought to be able to evacuate throughout the night. It's ridiculous that they shut us down at five," I said.

"They said that they're coming back first thing in the morning to finish the evacuation. We're being ordered to evacuate the facility by tomorrow, and we can't stay any longer."

"We'll gladly comply," I said. "What kind of order is that? What do they think? We want to be here?"

"The trooper wanted everyone lined up and ready to go right at daybreak," John said.

"Okay. We'll get the people off the helipad for the night since there won't be any more helicopters for the rest of the day."

I left for another trip to the pad but changed my mind, feeling that I needed some time to myself. I walked over to the edge of the ramp leading to the water. The frantic chaos of the evacuation from here just an hour earlier had dissipated like smoke in the air. Leaning on the brick wall, I gazed out alone over the murky, gasoline-tainted water, wondering when the nightmare would end. One of the staff doctors walked over to me.

"Richard, how are you doing? Really," she asked.

"I don't know. I suppose all right," I said. "I just don't know where my family is right now. I don't know if they made it out." My voice surprised me as it trailed off and faltered toward the end of the answer. I lowered my head and turned away to avoid embarrassment. As tears ran down my cheeks, I walked a few steps away to be alone again and sobbed in silence.

As I started back through the hospital in the direction of the helipad, nurses, patients, and refugees stopped me and asked for information. People were desperate for reliable information. Rumors ran rampant throughout the hospital and filled the vacuum left by no information from the outside world. Rumors became fact as they resurfaced over and over. I tried to reassure people that the state police would be returning first thing in the morning to get everyone out.

"We done heard that before, Doc," an old man with swollen feet said.

"Yeah, no one be coming for us," the lady next to him joined in.

"We not gonna make it much longer in here, Doc," he said.

"Just hang in there for tonight and we'll all be evacuated by tomorrow," I said, wondering if my personal doubts about this didn't betray my attempt to give him some hope.

I broke the news to the group of about thirty who had been waiting all day on the helipad catwalk: No more choppers would be coming for the rest of the afternoon. They had grown accustomed to the disappointments. Everyone would have to leave the catwalk and regroup down below in the parking garage. Given the difficulty of moving people back through the crawlspace hole on the second floor, and the oppressive heat inside the hospital, the entire group would bed down for the night in the garage. We would bring them back down to the second floor of the parking garage, which served as a staging area for transport up to the helipad. About ten people were already there, waiting to come up. Betty and Paul began the demobilization from the helipad area, while I went down again for the evening crisis meeting.

On my way to the meeting, Dr. Skinner, the professorial pathologist, came up to me.

"Richard, we've run out of room in the chapel," he said, stroking his beard and peering over his glasses.

"So where are you putting the bodies now?" I asked.

"We are leaving them in their own rooms."

"It's better that way so that all the people don't see these dead bodies being transported through the corridors to the chapel. What's the death toll so far?"

"About eight or nine."

"That's more than we would usually have during normal conditions," I noted.

"Yeah, the terminal patients just aren't doing well. We don't have any body bags, and the chapel is starting to smell pretty bad. We're still wrapping the bodies in sheets."

"I'm worried we'll have more die tonight."

"I'll give you an updated number in the morning," he said.

The evening's crisis management meeting took place outside on the ER loading ramp. The meetings had steadily drawn fewer people as they either had other responsibilities or they didn't know when or where the meeting would be, given the lack of communications. I noticed that none of the maintenance department personnel were there. About a dozen people assembled just above the water line in the steamy conditions. All the airboat noise of hours before had vanished. The meeting was very informal and served as a chance to hear the hardships of other members of the team. The biggest problem we now faced was the lack of security.

Susan, our commander, standing above the crowd, gave the most recent developments. Most of the Baptist security guards had deserted and gotten out on the boats earlier that day. Only one NOPD officer remained. The lone National Guardsman had been pulled out earlier in the morning. Dave Goodson, the boyishly good-looking go-to guy, was off at the time with the maintenance workers and deputizing them.

"Susan, what do you mean, 'deputizing them'?" someone asked.

"They're being given a crash course in law enforcement," she said. "Dave's passing out guns to them and instructing them in how and when to use them."

The newly armed men would be posted at most of the entrances to the hospital from the water. They would set up a perimeter that would include just the hospital building itself. All the outside buildings would go unprotected. Many people, myself included, had been sleeping in sites outside this perimeter. The few civilian guards now available couldn't even guard all the hospital entrances well, much less the surrounding buildings. I wondered about the boatloads of looters I had seen the night before. Would we be next on their list? Should I sleep in the hospital somewhere?

Our plan was once again to have everyone ready to go first thing in the morning. The state police had assured Susan and John that they would resume the boatlift shortly after daybreak. They planned to bring larger boats to speed the evacuation.

I gazed over the water as people talked in the background.

By now, virtually all the patients had been moved from their rooms to staging areas for evacuations that had not occurred. Many patients had been shuttled between multiple sites. The lack of a clearly defined nursing unit responsible for a patient's needs was one of many breakdowns in the delivery of care. Any semblance of a modern tertiary-care facility had now vanished. This wonder of modern medicine had no running water, no electricity, no elevators, and no telephones. The whir of the laboratory and radiology departments was another casualty. The hospital didn't even have a place for its dead. Now it was trying to defend itself against marauders who might attack in the night, with its own makeshift militia.

Many patients just lay on the ground. The nurses, staff, and volunteers made steady trips to the pharmacy to obtain the scheduled medications for patients. As the heat took its toll, the healthy patients were weakening. Older relatives and friends of patients were now getting weak and becoming patients in need of care themselves.

Moving patients on stretchers or wheelchairs up and down dark stairwells and corridors was extremely labor-intensive. Hundreds of non-medical evacuees had volunteered to perform many chores, including feeding patients, getting medications, running messages, transporting patients, carrying supplies, and fetching water. This small army of extra help was now losing its collective strength as its members wore down.

I could feel myself getting weaker, too. My belt was already notched up by one hole since Sunday. That seemed so long ago, now.

What was life like back then? I wondered if I still had the strength to swim out of here and walk to safety if it came to that. *Stop thinking that stupid stuff,* I told myself, *and get back up to the helipad to get those people down.*

On my way to the crawlspace leading outside to the helipad, I witnessed dozens of people sprawled on the floors and corridors of the hospital, lifting their voice to ask for water and assistance. The sun was now near the horizon, but it had baked the building all day, and the heat was unbearable.

I got out through the crawlspace and onto the parking garage. The group of about a dozen people waiting in the staging area on the second floor of the garage had swollen to about twenty people, as those from the helipad above slowly migrated down.

Those who could walk had hiked down the circular parking garage ramps down to the second level. The Magnolia garage transport service kicked back into gear, too. A black pickup came up to the top level, and volunteers loaded people into the bed of the truck who were too weak to walk. The truck then brought these people to the campsite on the second level, unloaded them, and went back up to repeat the cycle again.

The second floor of the parking garage was littered with excrement of all kinds. The animal kennels were in the garage, where hundreds of owners walked their animals. Every step ran the risk of landing in dog shit. Humans took dumps between the parked cars. Human and animal urine puddled on the level parts of the concrete and dribbled down the ramps in small, yellow streams. The area smelled like a cesspool. But the conditions here were better than those inside. I found a place where the density of stool clumps was low, and claimed it for our makeshift nursing unit for the night. I kicked a few of the remaining turds out of the way.

We needed things to make the place halfway livable for the night. I brought a five-gallon water jug to the improvised campsite and set it up with cups. The cook had put together some crackers, a mysterious cheese spread, and some canned fruit for the evening meal. The serving line for this feast was inside, so some staff members went over for the food and brought it back. I put together a team to go on a scavenger hunt for mattresses and pillows for people to bed down with on the foul concrete. The team of seven or eight of us made two trips into the dark, hot hospital corridors and searched each hospital room for things that we could use at our makeshift nursing unit. We eventually scored about thirty mattresses, pillows, and sheets for everyone.

Once the mattresses and pillows were arranged, the patients lay down to rest for the night. The constant barking of the dogs, the raw sewage smell, and the humid conditions would make sleep difficult at best. I knew that people wondered why they had trekked down from the helipad to sleep in these conditions. Morale was at a low point for the nurses, patients, family members, and evacuees. Maybe another one of my periodic updates might help to bolster spirits.

"Hey, I know y'all have been through a lot today," I started. The stench of the air and the barking of the dogs presented new distractions since my talks in the catwalk tunnel to the group. "We had to move down here since we didn't have enough room for everyone to lie down in the catwalk. Even though it's not that great here, conditions inside the hospital are a thousand times worse. It's definitely a lot better out here than in there. Anyone who wants to go inside for the night can go. We'll help you if you need help."

Not one of the thirty got up to go.

"When are we getting rescued?" an old man asked.

"We've been reassured that there'll be lots of boats coming first thing in the morning for us all. Being down here, we're closer to the boats now for when they come tomorrow. Be sure to drink plenty of fluids. The water is right over here. The staff can get it for you if you need them to."

"Doctor, my mother is here with cancer," a man in his sixties said, pointing to a feeble old woman on a mat at his feet. "She's in pain and can't even get a Tylenol. Nobody cares about us. You're not going to get us out of here."

"That's not true. We are doing everything possible to evacuate this place. If your mom is in pain, we'll get medicines for her," I said.

"We're going to die in here," he said.

"I don't want to hear any of that talk from you or anyone else," I snapped. "We're getting out of here tomorrow. It's true that people have died in here, but we're doing all we can for everyone. If you want to dwell on dying, go ahead. The rest of us are focusing on living and helping each other out so we can all get out safely. Don't give me any more of that talk."

He was right about the problem of getting medications for the patients. The usual mechanism of medication delivery from the inpatient pharmacy involved pneumatic tube delivery to the nursing station or delivery via a locked supply cabinet that was prepared in the pharmacy. Now a staff person or volunteer had to make individual trips to the pharmacy through the dark hallways to retrieve the medications for a patient. Multiplied by three or four doses per day and two hundred patients, hundreds of trips to the pharmacy were necessary to provide the medicines. The staff was exhausted.

Afterward, I went up to the man with the sick mother.

"I want to help your mom and to reassure you that I'll help her however I can," I said. "What type of medicine is she taking?" I picked up her chart and looked through it.

"She was taking Tylenol or Tylenol #3 for bad back pain," he said.

"I'll go down to the pharmacy and get some for her."

"Thanks a lot. I'm sorry I was upset and told you those things awhile ago."

"No problem. It's a stressful situation, no question."

I went back into the hospital through the crawlspace on the second floor. The pharmacy had no outside windows nearby. The only light in the area came from the dimming flashlights of the workers inside. I signed for some Tylenol and Tylenol #3 and went back to the parking garage. As I gave the lady her medicine, I was taken aback at how primitive the delivery of health care had become here in just four days.

Once the group had settled down for the night, I talked to the nurse who was overseeing the makeshift unit.

"Joanne, do you have staff to stay here with them tonight?" I asked.

"We're really worn out," she said. "You know when this thing hit, we had one full shift of staff working. Obviously, no one was able to come in and relieve us, so we've been doing the work of three shifts a day for four days straight. We've split the staff in two so that half the staff works a shift and the other half rests. They then take turns working. But, yeah, we'll have people for tonight."

Joanne and her team stayed on duty in the garage/kennel all night. Months later, she told me of an unexpected midnight visit by some law enforcement officer with a stiff, wide-brimmed hat. She wasn't sure what he was doing there or how he had arrived. She thought that maybe he had come to cherry-pick a relative, as others had done before.

He walked up to her amid the squalor.

"Ma'am, I've served in Iraq," he said to her. His brim was almost touching the top of her head. He paused. "This is worse than anything I ever saw over there."

He left as tears welled up in Joanne's eyes.

After nightfall, I walked around the unit's perimeter to check on security. A maintenance-worker-turned-armed-guard sat in a chair near the end of the car ramp as it disappeared into the black water. The water gently lapped at the cement embankment as he watched and wondered. At the other end of the garage, an unguarded stairway descended into the water. I decided to stay and help secure the area until I didn't see any more looting going on from the boats below. I didn't have any way of preventing such an attack, other than serving as a fierce-looking decoy. That would have to do.

Looters traveling out by boat that evening roamed the neighborhood and returned with their boats filled with TVs, stereos, clothes, and other goods. I had no problem with looters going to go get food and water, but I was completely disillusioned that they would use this opportunity to steal TVs and things that didn't even work at the time. Gunshots still rang out in the distance. We heard reports of mobs storming Meadowcrest Hospital and raiding the pharmacy. We knew we were even more vulnerable to such an attack. I prayed our newly trained militia was up to the task.

By around ten o'clock, all the looting activity outside the hospital had stopped. The security situation seemed relatively under control. I decided to go to my unsecured office building to get some rest.

I climbed through the small crawlspace leading back in to the hospital. Dim flashlights flickered at the opening of the small tunnel.

Voices echoed from the far side of the room filled with a huge tangle of water, gas, and steam pipes. Guided by my own dim flashlight, I stepped through the utter blackness toward the doorway leading to the second-floor corridor. The sounds of moans, groans, and gurgles wafted through the hallways. The heat was overpowering. About two hundred people were lying, sitting, and squatting in the dark halls. Nurses and staff were desperately fanning patients with their charts, magazines, or clothes. Sweat was everywhere. Volunteers sopped up the sweat from the foreheads of those scattered at their feet. People called out for water and pain medicines. The heavy, stuffy air was unrelenting in its oppressiveness. Most were too weak to escape it.

Dehydration was a killer for both the healthy and the sick in this situation. The armed guard sat next to the water dispenser at the end of a crosswalk, glass scattered about the floor. I filled several water bottles from the five-gallon jug, and brought water to some of the neediest. Many were already too weak to even swallow. The difficulty in getting supplies and the poor sanitary conditions made it impossible to provide IV fluids for everyone. Priority was given to those who already had IVs going. I discussed the situation with several nurses and doctors among the crowd. We would try to start IV fluids on those whose blood pressure was low.

The staff felt frustrated and helpless, with so many people suffering so much, and not being able to provide the care the patients needed. The lack of communications, electricity, and supplies had turned them from highly skilled medical caregivers to comfort-givers without much concrete therapy to offer. They knew that some would not survive the night, and the death toll would grow exponentially the longer they were stuck in this hell. I offered several patients the option of going to the garage. None of them wanted to leave the hell they were in for an unknown hell they might be thrown into somewhere else. Hope was fading.

"Hey, Richard," Larry shouted from the center of a crowd of patients lying on the floor. "What should we do with these people? It's too hot in here for them."

I was surprised to see him. The eye patch was off. His limp hair and forehead dripped with sweat. He was fanning a patient with a chart.

"What are you doing here?" I asked. "I thought you left on Tuesday."

"Didn't have anywhere to go and I didn't want to be alone," he said.

"Well thanks for fanning these patients and helping out. Try to keep them hydrated as best as possible. We can't start IV fluids on everyone, but use your judgment on who really needs it. Keep plenty of water around for everyone. It's less hot outside in the parking garage. You want to move anyone out there?"

"I'll see if anyone wants to go. They're pretty much too tired to go anywhere. In fact, we're all getting pretty worn out."

"I really admire your dedication to be doing this. How are you doing, anyway?"

"I'm tired, hungry, and thirsty. Just like everyone else. God, I hope we get out tomorrow."

"I think we will. Supposedly, the state police are coming with a bunch of boats. Do you need any water?"

"No, thanks," he said.

"I'm going back to the office to try and get some rest," I said. "Be sure to get some rest yourself. I'll see you in the morning."

I walked through the crosswalk over the glass shards on my way to my office. I passed the armed guard at the outer secured perimeter of our facility. The dark hallways of the unsecured building of my office spooked me at every corner. I reached my office, unlocked the door, and felt relatively safe inside.

None of the windows in the office had broken, and the heat had been accumulating *a la* greenhouse effect for four days. My dirty skin had layers of dried, salty sweat and who knows what kind of bacteria growing on it. Without running water, a shower was only a dream. I gathered two bottles of rubbing alcohol and several towels. In the faint moonlight shining in through an examination room window, I stripped off all my clothes. I next unwrapped the dirty bandages from the cuts on both of my hands. One of the cuts had healed. I noticed the other cut was red around the edges and, after cleaning it with alcohol, I re-bandaged the hand.

Turning my attention to the rest of my grungy body, I first rubbed my arms and legs with a towel saturated with alcohol. The alcohol felt cool to my skin, with just a trace of burning in some of the superficial cuts which had accumulated unnoticed. The towel was brown after the first pass. Using more clean towels saturated in alcohol, I eventually wiped off the grime on my back, chest, and abdomen. I can't say I felt clean, but at least I was disinfected. I put my dirty boxers back on and lay down on a clean sheet on the floor.

My last night in this hellhole, I tried to convince myself.

CHAPTER 5

Thursday

"Brownie, you're doing a heckuva job."

— President George Bush complimenting his FEMA Director, Michael Brown, on the rescue effort.

The crisis meeting began shortly after Thursday's sunrise on the ER loading ramp. The meeting started early, in anticipation of the flotilla of boats which would be arriving soon, so that no time would be wasted in moving people out. A faint morning fog hung low over the floodwaters. The physicians and staff chatted and strolled about. Some sipped from their water bottles; others snacked on a piece of fruit. Confidence and optimism hung in the still air. We were sure that this was the last day.

Susan and some other administrators arrived. Susan stepped up onto the curb of the ramp, slouched and with a frown on her face.

"Okay. Listen up everyone," she began.

The group quieted down to hear about the arrival of the boats and how we'd organize the evacuation.

"No one is coming. The state police told us they can't come for us."

The crowd of physicians and support staff was suddenly quiet. I wasn't sure I heard her correctly. The faces filled with smiles had now turned to somber, stern looks intensely focused on Susan.

"They told us we'll have to save ourselves," she continued.

I had heard her correctly, after all. They really weren't coming.

I was standing next to John as she spoke. Her statement had two opposite effects on me. The first wave of feeling was that of a body blow to the gut that had taken all the air out of me. I felt as if I would eventually breathe again, but I just didn't know when or how it would happen. The recurrent disappointments and neglect had almost made me numb to the news. But the next emotion I had was that of power and control. Finally, we absolutely knew we couldn't trust anyone to come get us, even if they said they would. We knew that our rescue was totally dependent on our own ingenuity and skills. No longer did we need to wait for someone else. We would begin to save ourselves using our own resources. The repeated promises of authorities that they were coming for us had undermined our ability to take the necessary steps we would have taken all along to get ourselves out.

"Tenet headquarters is trying to get airspace rights to send helicopters for us," Susan continued. "Eric and Dr. Casey are going to scout around in a boat to see where the dry land is." Glenn Casey served as the head of the anesthesia department at the hospital. He was tall, thin, and intense. He would go to the mat for an idea he believed in.

John and I were standing at the back of the crowd. John's unwashed black hair shined with five days of oiliness.

"Richard, we can't wait for Tenet to send in helicopters. If Glenn finds a dry route out, we have to evacuate ourselves," John whispered.

"I agree totally. We can't get fifteen hundred people out by helicopter."

"You need to take over this meeting and tell Susan how we're going to do the evacuation."

"I'm not going to do that. She's the leader. I'll talk with René after, and tell him you and I think we should focus on evacuating ourselves by boat."

"That's the only chance we have."

"Tell me what Glenn is up to," I asked.

"He took the only boat we have that wasn't stolen and is looking for dry land close by," John said. "We'll commandeer boats from around the neighborhood if there's a good evacuation route."

"If he does find a route out, we should move the entire group out and set up a field hospital there if we need to. We can boat supplies to the area and set up some kind of security perimeter. At least we'll be out of this place."

"Lots of people here could just walk to safety if they had the chance," John added.

"We could rely on local homes for food and water if we absolutely needed to."

While John and I were talking, the stunned crowd had regained its voice and people were shouting questions.

"How long will the helicopters take to get here?" someone shouted.

"Why won't the National Guard or state police come?" another queried.

"We can't last here much longer. We're short on food," an older doctor commented.

Then the winner of all: "If Tenet sends in helicopters, does that mean we can only send people to Tenet hospitals so they can keep the business?" Larry asked.

René walked over to me. "What in the hell is he talking about?" he moaned to me. I thought that if his Cajun temper flared up, Larry might need another eye patch.

"Like anyone is worried about whose facility we can get rescued to," I said.

We both rolled our eyes and he walked away.

After the group quieted down, I spoke. "I think our best bet is to get ourselves out of here on boats, depending on what Glenn finds out. It's a way we can rely on ourselves and give people some hope."

"We're going to just have to wait on them and also on what we find out from Tenet," Susan said.

More talk followed, and the meeting broke up. John joined Glenn on the scouting expedition during one of his passes by the hospital.

Before everyone dispersed, I caught up with Dave Goodson. Dave somehow had managed to maintain his squeaky-clean boyish face and neat hairstyle. If we were to start a boat evacuation, we would need fuel.

"Dave, we're gonna need lots of gas for the boats if we get this up and running," I said.

"True," he answered.

"Can you get some tanks together and siphon gas from the cars in the garages? We don't want to slow down the evacuation by waiting for fuel. Let's have the supply right by the dock."

"No problem. We'll get on it right away."

When Dave said he would do something, somehow he would always find a way to get it done.

I wanted to check on the group camped out in the crude nursing unit in the Magnolia parking garage as soon as possible. No one at the meeting knew anything about how that unit had done during the night. I hurried over to the garage and decided to track down René later. A quiet hung over the corridors in the early morning hours along the way. Throngs of people strewn about the floors stirred in their first attempts to face the trials of the new day.

Nurses with drawn, tired faces greeted me on the second floor of the garage. No one had died during the night, but one of the DNR patients, Mrs. Stevens, was barely breathing. I went over to her. Her fine, white hair lay limply around the pale skin on her neck and shoulders. Her eyes were closed and she couldn't respond to commands or to any sensations. Other than the feeble motion of her chest up and down, she made no movements. A slight gurgling noise came from her throat. How I wished for a suction catheter to at least suction her secretions. The inability to take care of even the most mundane problems was infuriating.

The group needed some information about the new plan.

"Let me have your attention," I said to the group. "We're making plans to rescue ourselves. The authorities aren't coming for us, and we aren't relying on them anymore. We know we can rescue ourselves, and will be planning on boating out to dry land. We have scouts going around right now, finding the best route out of here."

I really believed myself this time, and I think everyone else did too. After I answered questions from patients and staff, a flicker of hope reappeared in their eyes. My next missions were finding John to learn of the plan's feasibility, and talking with René.

Shortly after, John caught me in a hallway.

"Okay, what's the deal?" I asked.

"Glenn and I went all around. There's dry land up at Napoleon and St. Charles. What's even better is that you can drive a car from there all the way out to the Crescent City Connection and get across the river."

We suspected that there was dry land at the intersection about a mile away, since the state police and the Cajun airboat volunteers had sent people there yesterday. But we didn't know if it was surrounded by water and still cut off from a land rescue.

"That's perfect! If we can get everyone there, the healthy ones can walk out. The sicker ones can get a ride out," I said. I knew for the first time this plan was workable.

I went to find René. He was in a dark part of the parking garage when I caught up with him.

"René, John and I both think that we need to get ourselves out of here by boat and not rely on the choppers from Tenet. If they get here, great. But we can't wait any longer."

"How would it work? Where would everyone go?" he asked.

"There's a dry evacuation route all the way out of the city from the intersection of Napoleon and St. Charles. We can shuttle everyone out of here to that corner. We'll send supplies and set up a field hospital if we have to. A lot of the people here could walk to safety if we give them some food and water. Most of the healthy ones would definitely choose that option. That would relieve us of a big burden of feeding all these people when we don't have much food anyway. We could get food from nearby houses if we absolutely needed it. We'll set up a security perimeter. Hopefully, we wouldn't have to spend tonight there, but we'd be prepared to, if needed."

"Okay, I'll support that plan," he said. "Let's get moving on it, *cher*."

Up on the helipad, the team had already moved a group of people into position in the catwalk tunnel in case any random helicopters turned up. I brought Paul and Betty up to date with the latest news about the evacuation. Paul flashed those pearly white teeth when he heard the plan. Betty was ready to put her air force training to use up on the helipad. As we talked, a squadron of Coast Guard helicopters approached. The first one landed, and the commander said that they could take healthy people only. They could fly about an hour's worth of missions for us and then they had to go. It was our chance to evacuate as many as possible during that time.

Our healthy individuals waited in the catwalk and looked on as the first group of four or five of them boarded the helicopter. The voice chain down the stairwell sprang into action again as we called for more healthy people to come up to the helipad. We had initially devised the chain of voices the day before when the communications totally shut down. The chain of humans posted within earshot of each other stretched from the top of the helipad, down the many landings in the dark stairwell, and then out to the first floor of the hospital. This voice relay system provided the best means of communicating messages from one area to another. After filtering through as many as a dozen people, the message at the other end would often bear little resemblance to the original message, but without walkie-talkies, the scheme served its purpose.

By now, the helipad team had become very efficient in managing the helipad loading zone. The team always had an assortment of people to evacuate in the tunnel. Ambulatory patients, wheelchair patients, stretcher patients, and healthy evacuees stood by at the ready.

The most difficult patients to evacuate were those on stretchers. Few helicopters could take them since Acadian Air Ambulance had stopped coming. But if a chopper had the capability of taking a stretcher patient, we always had one or two of those available to go on a moment's notice.

For the next hour or so, the Coast Guard flew about twenty missions. We loaded each chopper in only a few minutes with about five people at a time. The pad had space for two choppers, and as soon as one was loaded, it took off and another would land. Captain Betty secured the landing zones so that no one would get hurt with the flurry of activity. The efficiency of our teamwork with the Coast Guard was impressive, and during the hour, we evacuated about a hundred people. Paul, Betty, and I all thanked the serviceman who helped us on the pad.

"I wish there was more we could do for y'all," he said. "Good luck to y'all. Maybe we'll be able to come back." He took off on the last chopper flight out.

In between the loud engine noise of helicopter landings, the sound of boat engines echoed up the building's walls from below. The silent sounds of death were now drowned out by the sounds of rescue. The tide of disappointment had turned. Like the excitement stirred up by the ear-jarring jangle in a casino, the sounds all around us finally indicated that we were on a winning streak. When the Coast Guard missions stopped, I left the helipad in the reliable hands of Paul and Betty so that I could help with the rescue efforts below.

I found John on a flat-bottom boat pulling up to the ER dock. His blue scrub top hung loosely on him, and the blue pants legs were wet to the calves. Eric, his upper body hulking over the motor, handled the controls at the back. Another flat-bottom boat idled nearby, ready to dock.

"Ahoy, Admiral Walsh," I said to him as he stepped onto the loading ramp. "You really got this fleet going."

"Yeah, we've rounded up all kinds of boats from the neighborhood," he said. "The only problem is that some don't have motors. We're just tethering those to the boats with motors. I'm having a blast."

John's boys had been commandeering watercraft of all kinds parked in the driveways around the neighborhood. The neighborhood's fishing fleet was now requisitioned for rescue duties.

"You obviously missed your calling," I said.

"There was one boat on a trailer. The only way we could get it afloat was to go under the water and puncture the trailer tires. It floated right off the trailer for us. One of the hospital electricians hot-wired it for us, and we were in business."

"How many boats do you have?"

"About six so far. We're still finding more."

"What's going on down by the drop-off point at St. Charles and Napoleon?"

"At first, nothing was happening. We only brought healthy people who could fend for themselves. Now there's more activity down there. The shuttle bus for the Audubon Zoo is picking up people and bringing them away. As more of us are gathering down there, more rescuers are coming to get us. There's a guy with a truck who's picking up people too."

"Can we bring patients?"

"The boats can only maneuver to within two blocks of the land. Then you have to get out and wade through about knee-deep water to get to dry land. If they can walk through that, they can do it. If they're in a wheelchair, someone will need to push them. The water would probably be right up to the level of the wheelchair seat."

"We just had a slew of Coast Guard helicopters up on top. They flew about twenty missions in about an hour for us."

"Yeah, I could see them all over up there."

"We still have about fourteen hundred people to evacuate, though," I said. "The Baptist Armada is definitely the way to go. I'm going to get a team together to staff and supply the drop-off point so we can get more patients over there."

"Good."

"Keep up the good work, Admiral," I said as I left.

I went to find Joanne, the charge nurse for our makeshift nursing unit, to assemble some nurses for the drop-off point. I found her still in the garage with the patients. The patients and staff wore weary smiles and spoke of the hope that today might be their last day here.

"Joanne, can I give you a big responsibility?" I asked her.

"You'll need to tell me what it is first," she said.

"We need to set up a unit on the dry ground at Napoleon and St. Charles. We'll need some nurses and some security. I'll take care of getting the security. But you'll be responsible for the patients and any supplies. You'll need food and water for people. You'll also need stretchers, wheelchairs, and whatever else you can think of."

"What's it like over there now?"

"I really don't know what you're going to find. You'll need to improvise as you see fit. There wasn't much activity at all before, but I hear that random citizens are just showing up to bring people away to safety."

"Okay. I'll do it. I'll start getting some staff and volunteers together now."

"Joanne, it might be risky. If you think it's too dangerous, just come on back. Send me back messages if you need anything."

"This is going to work, Dr. Deichmann. Don't worry."

"Go on down to the ER loading docks and tell Dr. Walsh to put you on the next boat when you get your team together," I said. "I'll let him know you're coming."

"Okay. I'll need to let Susan know I'm going off the facility, too," she said.

"I'll see you later."

I went up to the helipad to find Betty next. Betty's military background gave her the authority and experience to secure the drop-off point at the intersection for the evacuees. Betty wasn't there, but Paul was overseeing the pad. He told me that sporadic choppers had touched down, but nothing like the flurry of activity earlier. I told him that we might need to start sending people back downstairs to evacuate by boat if we continue to make progress by that route. For now, we wouldn't start making any changes, but I would keep him posted. He beamed his easy smile to me, and I knew he was good for any challenges that might arise on the pad while he was there alone.

Downstairs on the first and second floors was a beehive of activity. The crowds looked like the masses assembling to board the boats in the retreat from Dunkirk. The dock itself had dozens of people jockeying for position to be sure to get on a boat. The problem now was that there wasn't enough dock space to accommodate all the boats waiting to land. The boats without motors were tethered to the ones that had power. Most of the boats were sixteen- to eighteen-foot flat-bottom boats. Half the fishermen in Louisiana must own one, and plenty of fishermen apparently lived in Broadmoor. Each boat was packed with about ten people.

"John, you're really moving them out," I said.

"Yeah, we really need more dock space, though," he said.

"Look, we might be able to make a loading dock out of the ramp leading into the Magnolia parking garage. It would be really convenient since it's at the bottom of the helipad. We'd have the option of sending people out by air or by sea, depending on which route is fastest."

"Well, check to see if it's accessible by boat. There might be some underwater obstructions like parking gates or fences that would be in the way."

"Okay. I'll get on this boat right here and check it out."

I hopped down into the flat-bottom boat next to the ER ramp. A man with a dirty T-shirt and a camouflage cap crouched by the motor. A younger boy in wet jeans sat up in the bow.

"Hi. I'm Richard Deichmann," I said to the man at the controls.

"Hey, Doc. I'm Jim. That's my son, Bobby, up yonder," he said.

"We need to check out another possible landing on the other side of the hospital. It's a couple of blocks away. Can you take me over there and we can scout it out?"

"Sure, let's go."

We cast off from the brick wall at the ramp and headed up Clara Street to Napoleon Avenue. The boat turned right and slowly passed the front of the hospital. Given our luck, I anticipated running aground on a submerged car, fouling the motor on a submerged shrub, or impaling the boat on an underwater street sign.

"Man, I can't thank you enough for coming to help us," I said to Jim. "Where y'all from?"

"We came in 'bout two days ago from Texas," he said. "We seen y'all was having a lot of trouble over here on the TV. We thought we'd just bring our boat over and help out. We wasn't going fishing anyhow."

"Y'all came all the way from Texas?" I repeated.

"That's right. The thing is, they wouldn't let us put in once we got here. They tried to turn us around and make us go back. We wasn't coming all this way to turn back. We told the cops 'Okay.' Then just snuck our boat in somewheres else."

"Unbelievable. Where else have you been so far?"

"We were out in the East until today. We took lots of folks off the roofs over there. Seen some really awful things, too, Doc. Bodies floating in the water, dead animals. Really nasty smell with all that dead stuff."

"Man, I'm just glad you came over to help us out."

"Yeah, we heard this place was in bad shape. So we came over here next to help y'all. First thing we done was to help one of your buddies get hold of some boats around here. We rounded up a few for y'all."

"Yeah, I know. We rounded up some more and now we have so many, we need more dock space. Turn here at this street," I said, pointing to the right turn on Magnolia Street.

He turned down the flooded street and traveled about a block and a half. The entrance to the Magnolia garage was on the right, but a small fallen tree partially blocked the opening to the exit ramp. The main entrance was blocked by a gate. We moved the tree out of the way and idled into the garage. The cement ramp soon rose up out of the water. People could easily enter the boats from the driveway or from the curb next to it. The Texan had not encountered any underwater obstructions along the way. The ramp was closer to the corner of Napoleon and St. Charles than the other ramp, and would shave about ten minutes from the shuttle times. It looked like an ideal ramp.

"This will work fine. Let's get back," I told him.

He put it in reverse. The boat cruised back out of the garage. Five minutes later, we motored up to the original loading ramp. I told John that it looked like a good evacuation site. We could start evacuating all those who were waiting for helicopters from the Magnolia side of the facility by the new dock. The crowds on the emergency room side of the hospital would stay on that side to evacuate.

Although the state police had reneged on their commitment to get us out earlier, a few state troopers suddenly turned up unexpectedly. They brought just two small airboats, but every contribution to our fleet was welcomed. Two or three other troopers maintained order on the ER loading ramp among the throngs waiting to board. The momentum had finally turned in our favor. We had already evacuated three hundred people since we started our self-evacuation, and we were still cranking it up. I needed to find Betty to set up a secure, military-style perimeter at the drop-off point. That intersection might be where we would be spending the night. I wanted us to be prepared for the possibility.

As I looked through the dim corridors, Dr. John Skinner, our pathologist, came up to me. His gaunt face, with its gray-streaked beard, peered down at me.

"John, what's the tally?" I asked.

"We had about ten more deaths last night," he said.

"Look, we're going to get everyone out of here in the next few hours. I want you to assemble a team and go through every corridor and room in the hospital and make a log of all the deceased. Let me know what you come up with before you evacuate."

"Okay. I'll start working on it now."

What a grim chore that's going to be, I thought. John was used to working with dead bodies, but not many of his volunteers were.

On my way back to the helipad, I came across Betty standing stiff and alone in the parking garage.

"Betty, I'm so glad I found you," I stammered. "I want to ask you to help with a big job. We're evacuating everyone to Napoleon and St. Charles. I need you to set up a security ..."

"I've had it," she broke in. "I've been working day and night here and just can't give any more. I'm just not taking this kind of abuse anymore."

"What happened?" Something had thrown her out of kilter.

"I'm up on the helipad directing things," she started. "A woman doctor is wandering around on the pad. I ask her to clear the pad and she won't. So I ask her again. She walks over to me and says, 'I'm the doctor and you're the nurse. I'm not going to be taking any orders from you. Let's just get that straight.'"

"Betty, you're a captain in the air force. She doesn't know anything about running a helipad operation."

"You know that and I know that. But I've had it. I can't go anymore. You'll have to find someone else."

"All right. But Betty, I want to personally thank you for the unbelievable amount of work you've done. The efficiency of the flights this morning, the communications with the Central Crisis Command at the Superdome, the safety you implemented around the pad. All of it and more was thanks to you. So it's okay. Take it easy. I can get someone else. In fact, if you'd like, I'll get you on the next boat so you can finally get out too."

"I don't know. I'll probably stay around a little while longer," she said.

I shook her hand, not knowing if I'd see her again.

Back out on the garage, at the makeshift nursing station, I told the staff and patients that we would be opening up a loading dock not far away. I directed the group of about fifty people to make their way with me down the circular ramp to the water. As the group shuffled to the evacuation point near the waterline of the ramp, I went back up to the helipad to bring more people down if nothing was happening up there.

Paul, still with that confident smile, was standing close to the opening of the catwalk.

"Hey, what's going on up here? Where are all the choppers you're supposed to be calling in?" I said.

"I guess they blew themselves out this morning," he said. "We've had periodic flights since then, but nothing regular. People are baking up in here."

"A boat ramp is opening up right below us in the Magnolia garage. If there's not much activity up here, let's send people back down so they can get on a boat."

"Okay. But the people all the way up here should stay for now. It's just so hard to get them back down those steps. Why don't you bring down the ones in the staging area just below the helipad?"

"That'll work. I'll let you know about our progress down below in a couple of hours."

After the flurry of activity this morning, we had called for more people to come up to the helipad area for potential evacuation. About thirty people languished inside the catwalk, hoping for immediate boarding onto a chopper. Another fifty or so waited at the base of the series of steel stairways leading up to the helipad. These folks replenished the group in the catwalk as that group slowly got out on helicopters. The shade from the helipad above kept this area less miserable than up on top.

I informed the group below the pad of the available boat ramp eight levels below. Most of the group didn't want to leave and make the trek down to the bottom. The ones who did followed me down to the waterline. There they sat on the ramp's curb and waited some more.

I needed to tell John that we were ready to begin, and that he could send over some boats now that people were in position. I also needed to find Dave Goodson, the ultimate multitasker, and ask him to assemble a team to set up a security zone at the drop-off point.

The afternoon was just beginning. The heat, the lack of toilet facilities, and the steady accumulation of fatigue hammered at everyone without relief. I began to worry after Dr. Skinner's report about the ten deaths last night that the stress and heat may not be the only causes of deaths. Given the horrible conditions, what if some infectious agents were at work? Refugee camps were famous as breeding grounds for cholera. Hospitals were home to some of the most lethal, virulent, and resistant bacteria in the world. All of the careful isolation procedures to prevent the spread of disease in this facility had totally fallen by the wayside three days ago. Patients with all kinds of serious infections mingled in intimate, unsanitary conditions with everyone else. The use of this non-functional hospital as a refugee camp could be an explosive incubator for an infectious disease outbreak.

The euthanasia question popped in my head again. But the notion of someone going around euthanizing people seemed really far-fetched. The idea didn't even warrant any further exploration. The news of the increasing numbers of dead, while not surprising, made me even more determined to evacuate this hellhole.

The clamor of the hundreds of people on the first two floors of the hospital had intensified. People realized that this evacuation attempt was not just another false alarm. They finally had a very real chance of rescue. The mob of people pressed together at the entrance to the ER dock staging areas to be sure they got on a lifeboat before the *Titanic* sank.

I saw John ahead on the dock. He was talking to one of the troopers. John's worn-out face had a look of exasperation. Perspiration soaked the dirty scrub shirt, as drops of sweat fell from his chin.

"Doc, we'll be closing down this loading ramp at five PM," I overheard the trooper say.

The state policeman, his sunburned muscular arms bulging out through the standard-issue, undersized uniform shirt, peered down at John from his enormous frame. Given the many obstacles John had faced already in his attempts to evacuate the two thousand people stranded at the hospital, he now bristled at the latest obstacle that the state trooper was imposing.

"Officer," John said, "there's no way we'll be finished evacuating all the people by then. There'll still be plenty of light left by five. There's no reason for us to shut down our evacuation then."

"We just can't guarantee security around here after five." The officer swaggered, brandishing his sidearm and a twelve-gauge pump shotgun.

"Officer, we just don't see much of a security problem right now. Everyone in the neighborhood is gone or trying to get out of this damned place. No one is threatening us."

The trooper stepped toward John.

"Doc," he said. "We'll decide what are security threats and what aren't security threats."

"We can't spend another night here," protested John in his baggy scrubs. "A bunch more people will die."

"We're closing this down," the trooper repeated. "Five PM sharp."

"We're opening up a second evacuation route on the other side of the hospital," John said. "We've scouted this route. It's accessible to the boats and we might be able to get everyone out today if we have two docks working. We have a lot of people in staging areas on that side of the hospital, and it'd be easy for them to get to the landing we've made in that garage."

"You're not doing that either."

"What's the problem with that evacuation route?"

"We aren't going to provide security to that side of the hospital. And if you keep giving me trouble, we'll pull out of here completely right now. We're in charge here now. You'll be evacuating how we tell you to evacuate. Is that clear?"

John backed away. The trooper also turned away and went over to talk to one of his buddies.

We don't need your help now anyway, I thought. *Where were you when we really did need you last night? Do me a favor and just leave.* This was just another one of a million setbacks to be overcome. I stepped up and huddled with John to discuss how we should proceed.

"What's that all about?" I asked.

"Isn't that some shit?" John answered. "They just show up and start dictating how we're going to evacuate. They're just getting in the way now."

"We have all kinds of people lined up and ready to go from the other dock. I came over to tell you. We need some boats over there now."

"You heard the guy. He won't let us ship from over there."

"John, they don't have any cops over there to tell us what to do. They're only right here. I think we should just start evacuating from over there anyway. I'm getting everyone out of here today. They'll have to stop us by force."

"I agree. I'll send some boats over there now."

Before leaving the ramp, I went over to talk with the state trooper.

"Sir, we have to evacuate this place by today," I said, looking up at him. "We have almost twenty people dead inside right now. The only way we can evacuate by today is if we open another dock on the other side of the hospital."

"I already said you can't do that," he said. "You'll need to bring everyone from over there to this area for evacuation."

"It would take hours to transport everyone through that crawlspace back over here. It's just not practical."

"We're not providing security to that side of the hospital."

I detected just the slightest accommodation in his tone. It implied that he probably wouldn't bother us over there, but that he wouldn't do anything to help us either. The nuance was good enough for me. Besides, so what if I was wrong about his meaning? I intended to open up the dock no matter what he said.

Before I finally left the ER area, Captain Betty briskly stepped up to me. She was wearing an energized smile.

"I'm reporting for duty, sir," she announced. "What would you like me to do?"

"Cut it out. You really mean it?" I asked.

"Sure. I'm sorry I was so upset earlier. Everything had just got the best of me. I'm okay now."

"Well I would love it if you'd take up the task of securing the drop-off point."

"What's involved?"

"I'm not sure what exactly you'll find. More and more help is coming to bring the evacuees away. I heard that Acadian ambulances are showing up now, too. We need to set up a security perimeter around the whole area and maintain order among the evacuees as they board vehicles to be taken away. I haven't been there myself."

"Has there been any trouble so far over there?"

"Not that I know of. You'll need to enlist the help of some of the men once you get there. Tell them that I have authorized you to be the security chief of the area. What you say goes."

"Okay. I'm ready to get on the next boat out. I'll be back to get my stuff when it's time for me to evacuate."

"Good. Let Dave know that you've taken on the security duties at the drop-off site. Keep in touch and send back messages via couriers in case you need anything. Best of luck."

Her small frame wiggled through the crowd and boarded the next boat.

Meanwhile, I headed back over to the Magnolia parking garage to begin the boarding process. Along the way, I announced that another dock was opening up, and anyone who wanted to come over through the crawlspace could wait in the lines over there. A few dozen people followed me to the new docks. A nurse told me about two four-hundred-pound patients who they were having trouble getting down to the staging area from their rooms. Other than those two, it appeared that all the other patients were now in staging areas waiting to be loaded onto boats. After the new dock was up and running, we would work on the heavyweight transport problem.

By the time I got to the dock, the first boat was pulling up. An elderly, wheelchair-bound black lady waited first in line at the water's edge. We rolled a sheet underneath her while she sat in the heavy chair. Four of us then grabbed each corner of the sheet, lifted her up in the makeshift sling, and gently plopped her in the bottom of the boat. An orderly folded the wheelchair and stowed it safely in the bow. Two other ambulatory patients boarded while the boat's driver directed them to their places. Three more healthy evacuees then boarded, with instructions to look after the weak ones during the journey.

Variations of this exercise occurred dozens of times over the next several hours. I called for more people to hike down from the helipad and to walk over from the hospital as the queues for the Magnolia dock shortened.

As hundreds of people steadily left by boat, the facility was slowly becoming quieter. Dr. Skinner came up to me.

"Richard, I'm leaving soon, too," he said. "We went through all the floors of the hospital and have a log of the deaths. Nine bodies are in the morgue. They were there before the storm and are now under water. We counted a total of eighteen bodies elsewhere. As you know, after the chapel filled up, we kept the bodies in the rooms. I have all their names."

"So we have a total of twenty-seven bodies here now?" I asked.

"Yes."

"When you get out, get in touch with Tenet headquarters in Dallas so they can notify the next of kin and make arrangements to retrieve the bodies. These bodies are going to be a real mess if they aren't taken out soon. I'll keep tabs on any other deaths and notify Tenet of those when I get out."

"All right. Take care," he said.

"Thanks, John. Good luck," I said.

He disappeared into the crowd with his list of the dead.

The end of the ordeal was in sight. Only three or four hundred people remained. I planned to stay until the all the patients were safely on their way out, and then I would get on the next boat out. I needed to retrieve my few belongings in my office, if I was able to evacuate as I hoped. While I walked through the nearly deserted hospital complex, stragglers were casually smoking cigarettes in the parking garage.

"What are y'all doing?" I yelled at two guys leaning over a wall. "Get your stuff and get out of here. Now. We're trying to evacuate the whole place today. Get over to the boats so we don't have to waste time looking for you. And don't throw those cigarettes into the water."

"I didn't know we were getting out so soon," the one with the moustache said.

"Get moving down to the boats," I warned. "You'll get left behind."

Guided by my dimming flashlight, I made what I hoped was my last trek up to the eighth floor of my building. I packed a small bag with my laptop, water bottles, some leftover food, and batteries for my flashlight. There was no way to know what lay ahead, or any guarantee that I would get out today. And if I did leave today, I had no idea of where I'd be taken. Wherever I ended up, there may not be enough food and water. I tried to prepare myself, in case the future held another couple of days for me with no support. I then slogged out of my office in water-logged tennis shoes, back to the Magnolia loading dock.

The staff had finally figured out how to get the two four-hundred-pound patients down the steps. A series of plywood boards were now laid over the stairs, and the patients had used them as a slide to scoot down to the second floor. From there, the two big boys were transported by stretcher to the crawlspace. Spine boards were lashed together and supported the patients during transport through the crawlspace. Stretchers then transported them to the loading dock in the garage.

Both of them now waited in the queues at the edge of the water. We rolled the first one onto a large sheet of plywood to haul him into the boat. Eight of us lifted the edges of the board carrying the massive weight. Crack! The plywood began to split in half. We set the load down before the man fell through the middle and onto the cement. Nurses lashed two spine boards under the wooden board. This time the carrier held up. The man took up most of the space in the boat, which dipped deeper into the water as it bore the load and beached itself on the concrete ramp. Four of us rocked the boat back into the water.

"Thanks, Doc," the rotund man said with a weary smile. "I didn't know how y'all were going to get me out of here, but y'all done it."

I walked around the parking garage, rounding up more stragglers. An older person lay on a stretcher parked in between two cars. I walked over to get her and wheel her to the boats. My heart sank when I got closer. Mrs. Stevens's lifeless body lay there, abandoned amid the stench of animal feces and urine. Her pale white skin had lost what little color it had, and her thin, white hair lay matted on the stretcher. Her respiratory gurgles were now quiet. Her death was the first death I had personally experienced since the crisis started. I spent a few quiet moments with her, thinking that she had almost made it out. I pronounced her dead and then wrote down her name and birth date from her wristband onto a piece of cardboard lying nearby. I said a prayer and then covered her head with the dirty sheet.

Down by the water, boat after boat docked, loaded up evacuees, and sped off. Evacuees from the hospital came over through the crawlspace for departure. More and more people walked down from the helipad to get rescued. Helicopters landed periodically, but the lines by the boats moved much faster than those in the catwalk.

A group of three nurses walked down the ramp to me at the waterline.

"No one cares about us," shouted the thin one with the straight black hair.

"What do you mean?" I asked. "I care about you."

"We've been working here day and night. Now they're making us walk all the way back down here to get on these boats. They told us we were getting out by helicopter and to go up to the helipad."

"Well, we want you to be able to get out as soon as possible. The helicopters just aren't coming that often. This is the fastest way for you to leave."

"I can't take it anymore," she began to sob.

"Look, I'll get you on the next boat. Just come up to the front of the line here. One will be coming any second now."

The three of them went to get their belongings nearby. They returned and looked at the boat that was ready for them.

"That's it?" she asked. She swept her long, black hair out of her eyes and pointed to the flat-bottom boat.

"Yeah, let me help you in," I said.

"I'm not getting in that. I'll get my feet wet."

"You'll get your feet wet?" I lost it. "What in the hell do you think is going on here? We have people dying in here and you're worried about getting your feet wet? We've been waiting around for five days to get out of this damned place, and you're worried about getting your feet wet?" I could feel myself falling apart. "You don't deserve to be rescued. Let someone else get on this boat who wants to get out of here alive. Get out of the way."

She stepped away and several others eagerly jumped on board. The rest of her group looked at each other.

"Can we get on the next boat?" one of them asked.

"Yeah," I said, "but don't complain to me about getting your damned feet wet."

Five minutes later, all three of them took a step or two in the nasty water to board the next boat.

John walked up to me by the Magnolia docks to help with dock-master duties. His black curly hair was drenched in sweat.

"They've closed us down over there," he said. "We're bringing everyone else over here."

I looked at my watch. It was a little after five o'clock. I felt like Cinderella at midnight. The ball wasn't ending yet, not if I had anything to do with it. We still had about twenty patients to get out and about two hundred people to evacuate. But the state police were closing in on us.

"We're going to keep evacuating until they force us to stop,"
I told John.

"Go for it."

"Once we get the patients out, let's try to get on a boat and
evacuate together. Hopefully we can both end up somewhere that
has cold beer."

"You got that. I'll come looking for you."

We kept on going. But about forty-five minutes later, the
state police boarded one of our boats with shotguns and made it
turn around. The ball was over. The rest of the evacuation would
have to rely on helicopters alone for the last fifteen patients, one
of whom was the other four-hundred-pounder.

Weary walkers trudged back up to the helipad. The Baptist
limousine service cranked back up. Wheelchair and stretcher
patients were loaded on the back of the pickup truck again
and driven up the garage ramp to the area just below the
helipad.

Dave Goodson made another sweep of the facility to be
sure everyone from every nook of the hospital and its many
buildings was out and up on the top of the Magnolia garage. I
was amazed that he still had not a hair out of place. Helicopters
were landing more frequently now. Tenet had arranged for an
entire Texas helicopter company to fly missions. The fleet of
helicopters arrived, and choppers landed at a steady pace.

Captain Betty had made it back from her duties offsite,
and mingled with some friends on top of the garage. I had
been worried that the abrupt cessation of the boat shuttles
had left her stranded away from the hospital without her
stuff.

"Betty, I'm glad to see you," I said. "I thought you got stuck
over there when the boats stopped."

"I knew they were about to stop them, so I got on the last one
back to the hospital," she said. "I needed to get my bag."

"What was it like over there?"

"Things went pretty smoothly. Acadian ambulances actually started coming and backing up as far as they could into the water. We could pretty much load people directly from the boats into the back of the ambulances."

"Excellent."

"A guy with a flatbed truck brought lots of people over to Causeway and I-10. We didn't have any trouble with security."

"Everyone's got a ride out of there for tonight? No one will be stuck there by themselves tonight, right?"

"No," she said. "There won't be anyone spending the night out there on that corner tonight."

"Betty, thanks so much." I gave her a big hug. "At the pace of these choppers, it looks like we'll get the rest out in the next couple of hours."

"I'll be so glad to get in the shower."

I rounded up the last ten to fifteen patients and directed them to the catwalk. Two more elderly men had died while waiting in the staging area in the shade just below the helipad. Both men looked to be in their eighties. Their pencil-thin arms and legs lay lifeless at their sides. They might have made it if the state troopers had not closed down the boat evacuation early. An ambulance might be rushing them to a working hospital by now. I scribbled their names and birth dates onto the crumpled cardboard which held Mrs. Stevens's name. Then I covered their heads with the wrinkled, dirty sheets draped on their stretchers.

Our numbers steadily diminished as the afternoon sun dipped low. Paul managed the landings and triaged people onto the choppers. Only about a hundred people remained, including maybe a dozen patients. Unless the helicopters stopped coming, we would all be out by tonight.

As the last of us congregated near the helipad, Special Forces agents in black shirts began to materialize out of nowhere. All of a sudden, men with steely eyes and automatic weapons swarmed the upper levels of the garage and helipad.

It was nice to have the protection, but a little late. The men took up defensive positions around the perimeter of the garage, pointing their weapons toward the dark waters below. When I waved to one of the men and said, "Hey," I got an icy stare. The muscle-bound man turned away and scurried to his next checkpoint. I had the feeling that he would just as soon shoot a person as light a cigarette.

I finally took off my wet shoes and sat down next to John against the warm cement wall of the garage.

"John, we did it," I said.

"It's the greatest thing I've ever done," he said. "I mean it. This is what we went to med school for."

"I don't know if I'd go that far. We didn't really need to go to med school to do many of the things we did. There wasn't a lot of high-tech medical care, if you know what I mean."

"But, you know, we're doctors because we want to help people. I never helped so many people at once in my whole career. It was great."

"I wouldn't want to do it again. It was good helping everyone, but I think it's been a pretty awful experience."

"We'll need to get some beer when we get out of here soon."

"Definitely. And there needs to be plenty of it and it needs to be plenty cold," I said. "Let's try to get out together on the same chopper, since we don't have any boats to get on."

"I might be leaving soon with Glenn. Supposedly some cop is going to come by boat to get him," he said.

"I wanted to leave by boat, too, since we arranged that whole thing, but I want to wait to be sure all the patients leave. I'll wait around awhile. We're pretty close now."

"If I don't get on a boat with Glenn, though, let's fly out to the nearest bar."

"You got it, brother." I pulled out a camera and took a picture of him, and wandered off to get a picture of Betty.

Up on the helipad, only a handful of patients remained in the tunnel. The last four-hundred-pounder was on a stretcher in the catwalk queue. I thought of the Herculean effort it had taken to get that man up to the helipad.

"Hey, Paul. Will any of these choppers be able to carry the big guy out?" I asked.

"Yeah. I got a special helicopter coming for that guy, one that can carry more weight," he said. "It should be here soon."

I talked to some of the administrators. They had done a good job, considering the situation they had been given. Things would never be the same again, in ways none of us could even begin to imagine. No one knew when or even if we would ever see each other again.

Awhile later, I looked around for John. A nurse told me he had left on a boat with Glenn, the intense anesthesia chief. I hung out in the tunnel as the line for evacuation continued to dwindle. About the only people left were the upper-level administrators and staff, a few physicians, and the holdouts with pets who weren't leaving them behind. The big boy also waited.

"Any more patients?" Paul called out. "Any more patients. Get on board."

Four men lifted a stretcher patient into the chopper, and a thin, elderly woman in a hospital gown stood next to the door. A larger helicopter for the big boy approached the hospital in the distance. Baptist was finally discharging its last three patients.

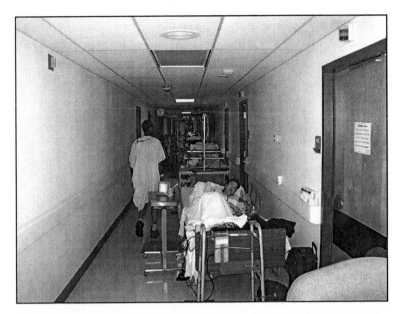

Patients line the corridors on Monday after Katrina blew out windows in the rooms. By Tuesday night, these corridors became pitch black when the generator failed.

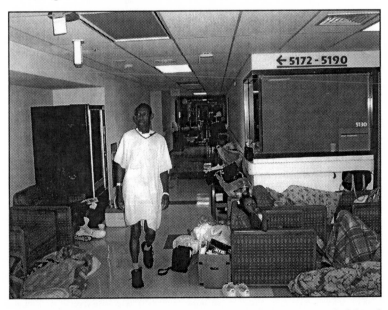

A patient strolls through one of many corridor campgrounds Monday while the generator still worked. The conditions were crowded, but relatively comfortable.

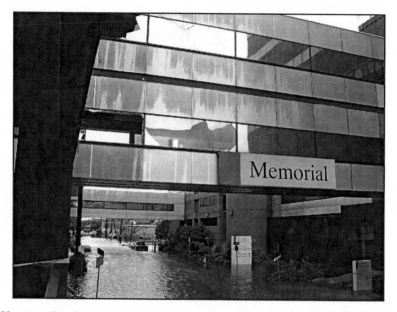

Katrina flooded the street and structurally damaged the crosswalk. By Monday evening, this water receded, only to be followed Tuesday night by eight feet of water from the levee breaks.

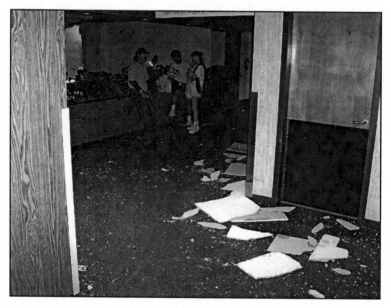

Ceiling tiles and shattered glass litter the water-soaked carpet on the second floor.

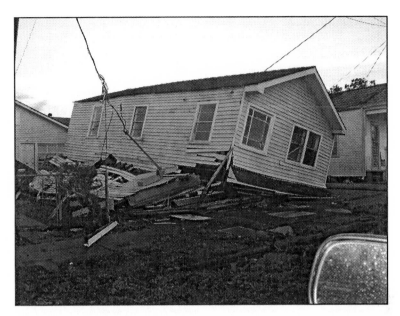

We saw this former two-story home from our car on our failed attempt to drive home on Monday evening.

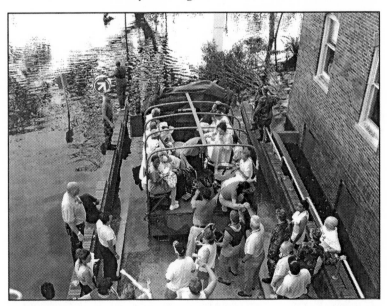

A National Guard truck evacuates a group of patients on Tuesday morning. The next truck stalled in the rising water about two blocks away, bringing the ground evacuation to a quick halt.

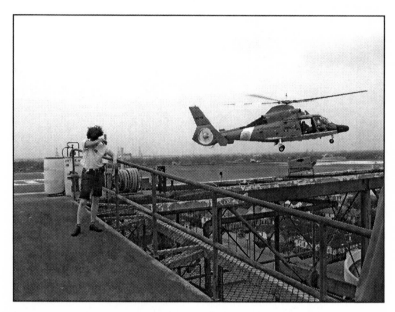

Captain Betty Bennett shields her eyes as one of the dozens of Coast Guard missions to the Baptist helipad departs.

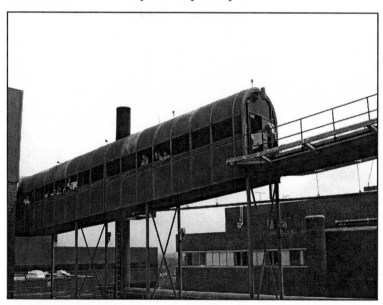

Patients and staff hang out by the broken-out windows to escape the ferocious heat of the catwalk tunnel leading to the helipad.

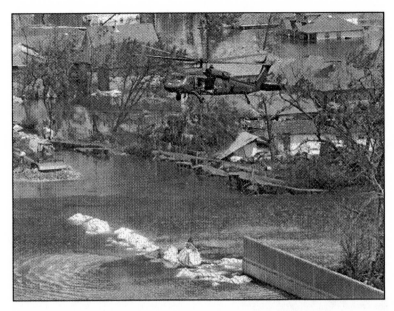

Water pours through the break in the Seventeenth Street canal levee. The earthen base of the levee gave way when the water level was still four feet from the top of the cement barrier.

From the Independent Levee Investigation Team report.

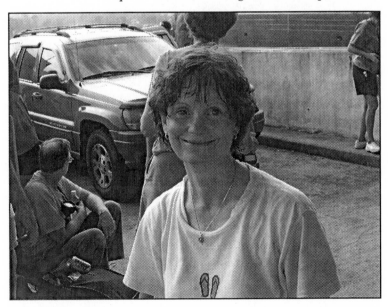

Captain Betty Bennett shows her relief late Thursday afternoon. The ordeal is almost over. She and I would evacuate about two hours later.

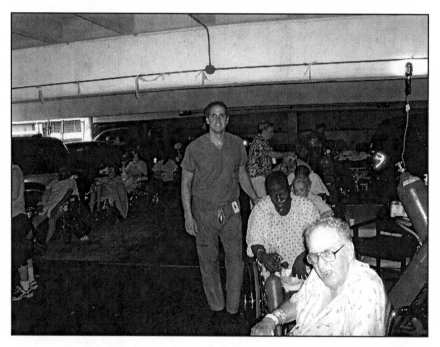

Dr. Bill Armington assists a patient waiting in the Magnolia parking garage near the evacuation boat ramp on Thursday. In the background, a nurse wipes the sweat from one of the many patients suffering in the heat.

Some patients died waiting in queues for evacuation. We notified authorities that people were dying in the hospital. The federal and state response was to close the airspace to prevent outside helicopters from landing and to restrict outside boats from entering the flooded area to help us. Four days after Katrina, the state finally told us they were not coming and we would have to rescue ourselves.

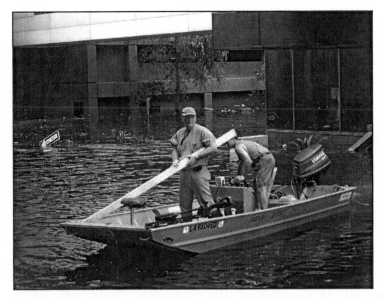

Dr. John Walsh and Eric Yancovich maneuver the flat-bottom boat toward the Baptist Hospital emergency room loading ramp to pick up evacuees on Thursday. The water is eight feet deep, almost submerging the street sign in the background.

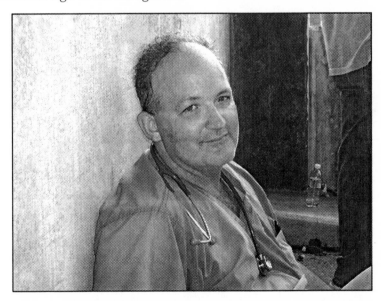

Dr. John Walsh relaxes late Thursday afternoon on top of the Magnolia parking garage after helping to evacuate more than two thousand people from the hospital.

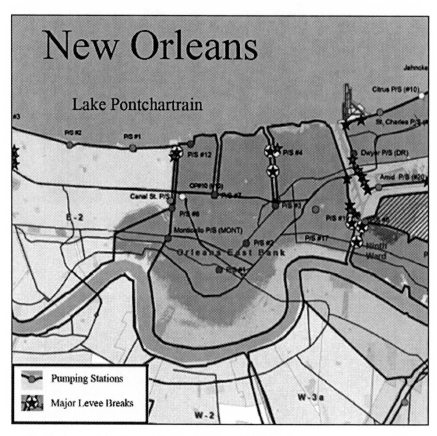

The Independent Levee Investigation Team documented the fact that the flooding was caused by poorly designed and constructed levees. Their report brought about improvements in the way the Corps of Engineers approached levee repairs and construction.

From the Independent Levee Investigation Team report, as modified by Jeff Jennings.

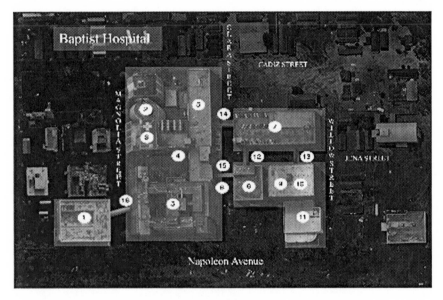

Baptist Hospital

1. Operating Rooms
2. Magnolia Street parking garage
3. Helicopter landing pad
4. Catwalk
5. Main hospital building
6. Emergency room
7. Jena Street parking garage
8. McFarland Building
9. Napoleon Medical Plaza
10. Dr. Deichmann's office
11. Cancer Institute Clara Wing
12–16. Crosswalks

From NOAA as modified by Jeff Jennings.

CHAPTER 6

Exodus

As you stand on the banks
You know you are so evasive.
Throw me a lifeline.
Save me! Oh, save me. Save me.

— Charmaine Neville from "save me"

"Okay," Paul yelled out, "we have room for two more people."

No one made any effort to get on board the chopper. Those who remained weren't ready to commit to leaving without a friend, colleague, or pet.

"Come on. Let's go. We have two more spaces," Paul shouted again.

I turned to Betty. "Let's leave together right now," I said. I thought how fitting that the air force captain was evacuating by air instead of water.

"Let's go for it," Betty said.

I walked out to the roaring chopper almost in disbelief that my turn had finally come.

"Hey, it's Dr. Deichmann," someone yelled. The small crowd in the tunnel clapped and cheered as I walked out to the chopper.

Their appreciation choked me up. The recognition caused me to think back on all we had accomplished and on the hardships we had overcome.

"Paul, the heavy guy is still back there," I yelled as I approached the helicopter. "You sure he's taken care of?"

"Yeah," Paul shouted back. "Get on this chopper right now. His is coming in to land right behind you. We needed to get a bigger chopper for him. Don't worry about it."

I looked up and saw a large military chopper getting ready to land.

"Thanks, Paul, for everything you've done. We'll have to get together after this is all over."

"We'll be talking about this for a long time to come. I'll get in touch with you."

I got in the chopper and sat next to Betty. The roar of the engines drowned out conversation. The copilot signaled to me to put on a headset dangling from a rack overhead. I put it on, looking forward to finding out where we were going and who were my rescuers. The headset was dead. *What else is new*, I thought. I couldn't communicate with them, and they couldn't hear me.

The chopper roared off the helipad and I was out of that deathtrap to points unknown. The pilot steered off to the northeast, as the sun hovered on the horizon to the west. Familiar landmarks passed below. City Park was completely inundated. The Fair Grounds was as totally flooded. Even from this altitude, the vastness of the destruction spread as far as I could see. The still shroud of death I'd witnessed from the top of the helipad was not a local phenomenon. Its reach extended for miles and miles, from horizon to horizon. A new sadness took over as the sun's last light flickered out. The blackness below had once been a city I loved. Now it was dead. How could it ever recover? No lights, no movement, no vibrancy. Soon, there was nothing at all to look at from the window. It was night, and the complete blackness made it impossible to pick out any landmarks.

I began to wonder where the helicopter would drop us off. Would we be dropped off at an evacuation center and left to fend for ourselves? Would they fly us to a hospital so the two patients with us could get immediate medical care? The chopper was still headed east, as best I could tell. Maybe we would go all the way to Pensacola, where I could recover on the beach. My thoughts soon turned to worry about catching up with Cecile and the kids. *Suppose they're still in New Orleans?* The thought was so horrible that I refused to acknowledge it. Assuming they had gotten out, where were they and how could I meet up with them? A lot would depend on where I was dropped off.

The thin woman in the hospital gown sat slightly slumped over in the third seat of the chopper with no emotion on her face. She wasn't happy. She wasn't sad. She was alive. That was good enough. I looked at the guy on the stretcher in front of us. His eyes were closed. His chest rose up and down in a strong, steady rhythm. He was a survivor, too.

I thought of a patient I had seen a dozen years before. He was lying in a bed in the intensive care unit on Thanksgiving Day after having had a series of strokes. The elderly man had a paralysis on his right side, swallowing problems, and speech problems from his stroke. His heart was in bad shape, and he was also battling a life-threatening pneumonia. I was checking his neurologic function by asking him questions to evaluate his mental status.

"Mr. Hebert, what day is it?" I asked.

"What you mean? What day it is?" he asked back with garbled speech.

"Well, what's special about today?" If he didn't know the day of the week, he might at least know it was Thanksgiving.

"Well, I woke up and I 'brothed,' didn't I? That's special enough."

Indeed, it was special enough to wake up and breathe for another day. The four of us in that helicopter shared and had a new appreciation for that most basic human bond.

The helicopter began descending into the darkness toward some landing lights in a sea of blackness. My senses were on high alert, searching for a clue as to where we might be.

A building came into view, along with some emergency vehicles next to the complex. The chopper touched down. Wherever this was had electricity—a major improvement over where I'd come from. The copilot got out and opened the doors for us. Nursing staff with wheelchairs and stretchers waited to assist. We had landed at a hospital of some type. I assisted the elderly black lady out of the chopper and a nurse took her off in a wheelchair.

"Where are we?" I asked an orderly.

"This is Northshore Regional," he said as he worked on getting out the remaining patient.

Northshore Regional Medical Center is a Tenet hospital in Slidell, a city northeast of New Orleans only about thirty miles from where I had been. This area had also been ravaged by Katrina, which had passed even closer to Slidell than to New Orleans. I was still not safe. Looking around, I saw the surrounding area was completely dark. Apart from the emergency generator of the hospital, no electricity powered the area. A bus was waiting in the parking lot next to the helipad on ground level. Betty was talking to a nurse over on the sidewalk next to the bus. I walked over to see what was going on.

"Dr. Deichmann, I'd like you to meet a friend of mine, Carol," she said. "Carol and I used to work together. She works here now."

"Hey, Carol. I'm Richard," I said.

"Y'all have really been through a lot," she said.

"Yeah. Thanks for taking us. It's been pretty rough. Is there a phone I could use inside? I still don't know where my family is."

"Sure. The phones are out, but we could see if they'll let you use the satellite phone for a few minutes."

"Great."

"Put your bag down here and we'll load it on the bus," she said. "The bus is taking everyone to Dallas, but it can stop in Baton Rouge if you'd like."

"Yeah, I'll probably want to get off in Baton Rouge. But if I can't get in touch with anyone, I'll go to Dallas." My sister lived in Dallas, but I dreaded the thought of a nine- or ten-hour bus trip through the night.

Betty, Carol, and I walked into the hospital. Carol brought me into the command center and introduced me to the doctor in charge. His saggy eyes and droopy face belied his energetic voice.

"Welcome," he said. "Glad to help you guys out."

"Thanks. What's it been like here?" I asked.

"We've been helping out with the evacuation some. But we don't have much staff, and everybody is overtired and overworked. We just don't have any relief."

"I can appreciate that. Hey, can I use a satellite phone? I need to get in touch with my family. I'm not sure they made it out."

"Absolutely. Try to limit it to a couple of minutes, 'cause we'll be needing it. None of the other lines or cell phones are working here."

"Thanks, and good luck to you," I said.

"Mike, show him how to use the phone," he said to a man with a button-down shirt, standing by a desk.

The man escorted me to the phone and I got Meredith's number out of my pocket. Meredith, Cecile's sister, was her closest friend and confidant. I knew it was no use to dial Cecile's cell phone. I had one shot to find out where Cecile was. If Cecile was in a place where she could contact someone, she definitely would have contacted Meredith. If Meredith had not heard from her, my worst fear would be true: Cecile, Claire, and Paige were still stuck in the death grip of New Orleans.

It was now about nine o'clock, Slidell time. Meredith, in Atlanta, might be in bed by now. If I couldn't reach her, I'd trek to Dallas to stay with my sister.

I dialed the number.

"Hello," Meredith said.

"Meredith, it's so good to hear your voice," I said. Tears welled up in my eyes as I heard her voice.

"Who is this?" she said.

"It's me, Dickie." She didn't recognize my hoarse, dry voice.

"Oh my God! We've been so worried about you. Are you okay? Where are you? I've talked to Cecile and they're okay."

"I've been so worried that they didn't get out. Where are they?" My voice was cracking and I didn't know how long I was going to be able to carry on a conversation.

"They made it to Lafayette, and are with Barry and Tricia and their family. Oh my God. I can't believe I'm talking to you. I love you. I was so worried." Now her voice was starting to crack. Barry and Tricia Breaux were our good friends and neighbors. They had offered their family's homes in Lafayette to us if we decided to evacuate.

"I only have a couple of minutes on this phone. I need you to get in touch with Cecile so she can come get me."

"Okay. Her cell phone's not working but I'll track her down somehow. I'll have to get her new number from Beth. She's been really worried about you too."

"Tell Cecile I'm getting on a bus to Dallas that's going to stop in Baton Rouge. I'm getting off at the Greyhound bus station in Baton Rouge. Ask her to meet me there."

"Suppose I can't get her?"

"I'll call you again once I get there to see what the plan is. I'm so glad to be getting out of here and to hear Cece made it out, too."

The man with the button-down shirt was looking at me with a half-scowl.

"Doc," he said, "you'll need to get off the phone now."

"Mer, I need to go. I'll call you when I get there in about an hour." I hung up and thanked the man for the help.

I walked back out of the room and down the corridors leading back to the bus. The bus had moved to a different position, but nobody was milling about. Betty was standing at the door of the bus and waving at me.

"Dr. D., get on the bus!" she yelled out. "We almost left you."

I sprinted to the bus door and joined her as she re-entered the bus.

"After we loaded your bag on board, the bus driver started to pull away," she said. "I noticed you weren't on and told the driver to stop."

"I can't believe I almost missed the bus. After all this, and then I miss the bus."

As soon as the bus left the hospital complex, complete darkness again enveloped us. No streetlights, no house lights, no businesses, no signs of life anywhere. Every once in a while, a lonely car would pass.

The bus was about half-full, with a hodgepodge of refugees from the city, both black and white, young and old. The worn-out faces all told the same story. Their tired saggy eyelids, rumpled up, dirty hair, and sunburned skin testified to the ordeal they each had suffered. Somber, quiet conversation drifted forward from the back of the bus. Our deliverance wasn't marked by wild laughter and celebration. We had seen too much tragedy. The enormity of it all was just sinking in. I recognized four or five people from Baptist who must have come over on a previous helicopter. We all had dirty clothes that smelled of five days of body odor.

Despite the appearances, I was in absolute luxury. The large, cushioned seats and the dry coolness of the air conditioning gave me the feeling that I was returning to civilization again. I reclined my seat back and planned to rest until Baton Rouge, usually about an hour's drive.

The blackness outside made it impossible to pick out any landmarks. The bus was traveling down some type of secondary road. When we started driving through a residential neighborhood after about fifteen minutes, I knew something was wrong. We should have easily been on the interstate by then. I started paying more attention to what was happening. We were driving around in circles in some subdivision. The bus driver turned around in someone's driveway. I got up and went to the front of the bus.

"What's going on?" I asked the driver. "Do you know where you're going?"

"I'm trying to get on the interstate," he said.

"Well, why don't you ask someone where to go?" Only three or four cars had passed us since we had left, so this would not be as easy as it sounded.

"I think I know where to go now."

"Okay." I went back to my seat, still not sure he knew where in the hell he was. After about another fifteen minutes we had still not found the interstate. When we came to the same intersection for the third time, I got up again and went to the driver.

"Stop the bus right here and let me off," I told him. "I'm getting out and getting some directions to the interstate from the next person that comes to this intersection. You don't know where you're going."

"Do whatever you want to," he said. He opened the door. I walked around to the front of the bus and stood near the driver's side. In only a couple of minutes, a red pickup truck drove up. I flagged it down and noticed two guys in their twenties in the cab.

The passenger rolled down his window.

"Hey, could you guys help us out?" I asked. "This is a bus full of evacuees from New Orleans. We're lost and can't get on the interstate to Baton Rouge. Could you give me some directions?"

"We'll do better than that, brother," the driver said. "Just follow me. I'll lead you right there."

"Man, thanks a lot."

I got back on the bus and told the driver to just follow the red pickup in front of him. They would lead us to I-12 west to Baton

Rouge. Five minutes later, we were cruising down the interstate to the Promised Land. Feeling confident that we were on our way, I snoozed in my regal setting. I dreamed of a nice shower and the comfort of a soft bed in an air-conditioned room.

The city lights of Baton Rouge disturbed my slumber. The bus now rambled along a city street, presumably to the Greyhound bus station. The delay at the beginning of the trip caused us to arrive later than expected. The bus slowed down to a stop in front of an old, dirty building that served as the bus station. Some of the houses and businesses in the block were boarded up. A small convenience store across the street was the only place open. Street thugs loitered in front. Garbage littered the street.

The dilapidated bus station in the middle of the ghetto was closed. A husky woman with a gun in her holster stood guard. The guard walked up to the bus after it had come to a stop. I got up to walk to the door. Five other passengers who were getting off followed me. The driver opened the door.

"This station be closed," the guard said to the driver.

"We have six people who want to get off here," he said.

"It don't matter. We be closed. They can't get off here." Her imposing body and massive buttocks filled the doorway and blocked the exit from the bus.

"Look," I said, "we won't go in the building. We'll just wait here for our rides."

"No. You can't be getting off the bus here. You gonna need to keep on riding."

Baton Rouge had already been inundated with refugees from the flood. I guessed that she had been told to not allow any more refugees to be dropped off in the city. That was her problem to deal with. I was too close to seeing my family to be turned away at this point.

"I'm getting off this bus right now," I declared. "You'll have to shoot me, but I'm getting off." I suddenly forced my way around her and the rest of the group followed. She was caught off guard.

"Y'all better not stand on this property," she volleyed back. "Get over there across the street. I ain't letting y'all stay here."

We got our bags from the luggage compartment and walked across the street to the sleazy convenience store. A pay telephone was stuck to a pole by the gas pumps. Some of my fellow evacuees got in an SUV that had come to meet one of them. But there was no sign of Cecile. Betty and I walked over to the payphone. I began to dial Meredith's number to see if she had made contact with Cecile. The SUV was loaded but didn't take off. A young guy with cornrows sticking out from under his black skullcap got out and walked over to me.

"Doc, you don't want to be hanging out around here," he said. "Trust me. We ain't leaving you here by yourself. Come get in the truck with us. We'll take you somewheres else."

"I think you're right," I said as I waited for Meredith to answer the phone. "Wait up for me." I quickly thought of some alternative site for Cecile to meet me, somewhere she had been before.

"Meredith, it's me again," I said as she picked up the phone. "There's been a change of plans. I'm going to the Embassy Suites off the I-10 in Baton Rouge instead. Did you get in touch with Cecile?"

"Yeah, she should be there by now. She's checking in with me every fifteen minutes. I'll try to call her again, but the connections aren't too good."

"Tell her not to go to the bus station. It's too seedy around here."

My pulse quickened, knowing that in only a short time, I'd finally be reunited with my family.

The cramped SUV pulled up to the valet area in front of the Embassy Suites hotel. Four of us piled out with our bags and thanked the driver.

Betty and I trudged inside. No sign of Cecile yet. Betty went to call her friend to come get her. I plopped down in a big chair in the lobby. The four of us stuck out like soup-kitchen bums at a dinner party, as we took seats in the elegant hotel lobby.

A few minutes later, Cecile rushed through the automatic doors toward me. Paige and Claire followed close behind. All three were wearing someone else's hand-me-down clothes that I didn't recognize. I got up and hurried over to hug them.

"You're all right. I missed you so much," I said to Cecile as I bear-hugged her. Claire and Paige stood on either side and just stared at their dad. I was gaunt, sunburned, dirty, and foul-smelling. My shoes still swished with water at each step. They weren't too sure they wanted me to hug them, but I did anyway.

"Paige, I love you so much," I said. "I don't ever want to leave y'all like this again."

I looked at Claire.

"Claire, you're okay? Let me give you another hug." She semi-willingly submitted. "I can't believe we're finally back together again. It's been so hard. I can't wait to hear what y'all have been through."

Barry, our neighbor, then walked through the hotel doorway, the typical spring to his step.

"I didn't know you were coming too," I said to him.

Barry grinned from ear to ear. His extended family had housed and supported Cecile, Claire, and Paige while I was missing in action.

"It's good to see you," he said as he bear-hugged me. "I'm the guy who brought everyone here. Come on, let's go. It's late and I'm parked illegally. We have a long way to go to get back to Lafayette."

I told Betty good-bye and introduced her to Cecile. Cecile and Betty struck up a conversation as they figured out that they knew each other from childhood days.

"Come on," Barry urged. "Let's go."

We climbed into Barry's minivan and soon crossed the Mississippi River on our way to Lafayette. Paige pulled out a bag of food.

"Here, Dad," Paige said. "I thought you would be hungry, so I made a sandwich for you. There's an apple and some candy too. Here's a drink."

"Paige, I am so starved. That was so sweet of you to think of this," I said as my voice began to crack. I was trying to contain a flood of tears.

"Tell me about your experience. I want to hear about that," I said between gulps of fruit juice. Listening to their story would give me the opportunity to avoid talking and breaking down in an emotional torrent.

Cecile, Claire, and Paige took turns filling in the pieces of their escape story.

After leaving the Baptist parking garage on Tuesday morning with a half tank of gas, they headed down Claiborne Avenue toward the Mississippi River Bridge. To conserve gas, they rolled down the windows and switched off the air conditioning.

After dodging road debris, they soon found the road completely impassable from rising water. To continue, the only option was to drive over the neutral ground next to a raging fire burning out of control on the other side of the street. A gas station had exploded, and flames shot high into the air. Cecile steered the car through the shallow part, with the flooded avenue to the right and the fire to her left. The intense heat from the fire beat against the exposed left side of her face. Another explosion at the station would have engulfed their car in flames. She kept going and made it through without the car stalling in the high water or exploding from the fire.

Once through this gauntlet, she traveled on, only to find that the entrance ramp to the bridge was under too much water. She'd have to find another route. She zigzagged her way through run-down parts of town, trying to find another approach ramp. Debris blocked the way at times. Flooded streets forced her to turn around at other times.

"Don't be going down that way," a local resident yelled out to her from the broken sidewalk. "It be flooded."

"How can I get on the bridge?" Cecile yelled back.

He answered, but his speech was so foreign, even Cecile, a native, couldn't understand him. Was he even trustworthy? She steered the car down the street anyway, only to find that the man was right. High water and debris blocked the road, and she turned around.

She passed the same man on her way back out to where she had started.

"I be telling you don't be going down that street," he said as Cecile drove by.

Relying on instincts to head in the direction of Tchoupitoulis Street, Cecile drove toward the river. She drove around in a maze of streets blocked by trees, power lines, or standing water, wondering if she'd ever find the way out. Suddenly and unexpectedly, she saw an entrance ramp to the bridge near Tchoupitoulis Street. Minutes later, she was on the other side of the bridge, with the dying city behind her. She had saved herself and her children. Now she needed to find her way to Lafayette.

They headed down Highway 90 toward Lafayette without a map. Cecile had never been this way before, but had heard that it led to Lafayette. Without any traffic on the road, they made great time through the heart of Cajun country. Cecile worried about what she would do once she got to Lafayette. Paige and Claire had been unable to reach Tricia or her daughter Lanie on the cell phone. Cecile knew they were staying with either Tricia's or Barry's parents, but didn't know the addresses or telephone numbers.

To compound her anxiety, the car was running out of gas. Since leaving New Orleans, she had looked for a gas station the entire way. She had traveled more than a hundred miles, and not a single gas station was operating. They were now close to Lafayette, and if they didn't find gas soon, they'd be walking the rest of the way.

Finally, with the fuel gauge hovering on "E," Cecile spotted a truck stop with several cars and eighteen-wheelers outside filling up. She pulled in and filled up. She was making progress; one less problem to worry about.

The kids got out and went inside to check out the junk food. Cecile joined them after topping off the tank and parking the car. She figured it was worth a try to contact Tricia or her parents from here using a land line. She went to a payphone and asked the manager for the phone book. She looked up Tricia's parents' name, Thibodeaux. Hundreds of entries were present. Same with Barry's parents' name, Breaux. It was like looking up "Smith" in an Anywhere, U.S.A. directory. That wouldn't work. She dialed the cell phone number again. Maybe now that services were better here, the cell phones were working. No such luck.

Cecile had one more idea. Maybe the truckers, with their fancy communication devices, might have a working connection. She walked up to a table with two burly truckers drinking coffee and smiled.

"I'm from New Orleans. I'm trying to get in touch with my friend in Lafayette, but my cell phone won't work," she said. "Do y'all have a phone that might work?"

"Sure, lady, you can try this one," said the one with the big tattoo of a naked woman on his arm. He handed her his phone.

She dialed the only number she had, but still no success. She gave the phone back along with her thanks to the tattooed man. Cecile, Claire, and Paige then got back in the car and headed the rest of the way to Lafayette, not quite sure what they would do once they got there.

By the time they arrived in the city in the early evening, the heavy traffic in the city turned every intersection into an exercise in patience. Tens of thousands of people from New Orleans had evacuated to Lafayette. The town was ill-equipped to deal with the massive influx. Cecile doubted any hotel rooms were available and thought that they may have to keep on driving. Before making any more decisions, they all decided to eat supper and try to figure out what to do then. They had not enjoyed a legitimate meal in days. Cecile pulled into a restaurant called Don's Seafood. They were seated after a short wait, along with Spice the cat.

"Hey, maybe I can text-message Lanie," said Claire, the cell phone expert.

"Give it a try," Cecile said.

"WE'RE AT DON'S. HELP," she punched into the cell phone. She put it away, not expecting any success, as usual.

Seconds later, the phone made its quirky sound. Claire looked at it. "STAY PUT. WE'RE COMING." Her eyes popped out, wide open.

"It's Lanie. They're coming over!" she told Cecile and Paige.

By the time they had finished eating, the Breaux family had arrived. Their deliverance was complete.

Their story finished, I had gobbled up the last bits of food in the bag. Now together once again, we approached Lafayette at the midnight hour. The Breauxs had arranged for us to live with Mrs. Thibodeaux, Tricia's mother. She had warmly opened her home up to Cecile, Claire, and Paige since that Tuesday night when they came over from Don's Seafood. We showed up in her driveway in the middle of the night, but she got up to greet us.

"Just make yourself at home," she said. "I'll just try to stay out of your way."

This was her house and she was offering to stay out of our way. Her generosity was overwhelming. She showed me the bathroom and bedroom. Before she went to bed, she gave me some clothes she had received for us as donations from her relatives. The life of a refugee was rapidly gaining meaning to me, as I realized that I didn't have any clothes of my own. She left to go back to bed.

I walked over to the bathroom to clean the filth off my body. The bathroom scale showed I was ten pounds lighter than a week ago, and now weighed a measly one hundred and fifty-two pounds. I showered, put on my secondhand boxers, and a red "Judice Inn — Best Hamburgers in Town" T-shirt, and collapsed into bed. But some unfinished business at Baptist Hospital trailed my thoughts as sleep whisked me away.

CHAPTER 7

The Aftermath

> *"When did we begin to lose faith in our ability to effect change?...You, along with the entire world, saw the bureaucratic fumbling and lack of concern inflicted on...citizens at the Superdome and the Convention Center. Who is being held accountable now?"*
>
> — Wynton Marsalis addressing Tulane students on Martin Luther King Day, 2006.

I awoke from an intoxicating sleep on Friday morning, knowing two tasks from yesterday still required action. Someone needed to be notified about the dead bodies left behind in the hospital. I was even more passionate about the other problem. The rescue effort by the civil authorities was a failure, but I felt that relatively simple steps could be taken to improve the effort and avoid more deaths. I had to talk with someone in authority.

I enjoyed some coffee and a bagel with Cecile before everyone was up and stirring about. I talked with her a little about some of my experiences. She brought me up to date on what she had been dealing with. I still didn't feel like I was back in real time again.

"Dickie, I know you've been through a lot," Cecile said. "But we need to live in the real world again and make some important decisions. Fast. Like where we're going to live, what school the kids should go to, how are we going to get jobs. Small stuff like that."

She told me of the lack of available housing in the area. No apartments were available for miles around. Many people were buying homes immediately, just to have someplace to live. She had visited a couple of schools and put Paige and Claire on a waiting list at one. Labor Day was in three days, and the kids would need to start the new school the next day. She had not even started thinking about jobs in the area, but that didn't look very promising. Both of us were out of work at this point with no income.

"Cecile, I need some down time," I finally said. "I just can't deal with all this right now. You may have to just make all the decisions. I'm decisioned-out."

"I can't make all these decisions," she said. "I've been waiting for you so we could decide together. Let's try to talk later today, then."

"Okay." I went over to turn on the TV to veg out and watch what was going on in New Orleans. I hadn't seen any television since Monday, and had missed the gory coverage of the catastrophe. After watching only a couple of minutes of desperate people still stranded on rooftops, looters in the streets, and helicopter rescues, I began sobbing uncontrollably. I turned it off and went back to my room, where I slept for another couple of hours.

My second awakening brought renewed commitment to reporting the deaths and making rescue recommendations.

I eventually got in touch with Tenet headquarters in Dallas and spoke with Michael Arvin, one of the chief administrators involved with the Baptist evacuation.

"Mr. Arvin, we have thirty bodies that are still at the facility," I told him after introducing myself to him. "Nine of the bodies are inundated in the basement morgue and were there prior to the storm. Dr. John Skinner, the chief pathologist, has the names of twenty-seven of the bodies. Three people died awaiting evacuation after he left. I have their names and birthdays."

"Let me get those from you," he said.

I gave him the names and told him that Dr. Skinner would be calling in with the log of all the other bodies.

"Most of the deceased's relatives probably don't even know about their loved one's death," I continued, about to erupt in tears again. "Be sure to inform the next of kin and retrieve the bodies so that proper funeral services can be arranged for. It's so hot in there, I'm sure the bodies are decaying really fast."

He thanked me for the information, and I gave him my telephone number at Mrs. Thibodeaux's house before hanging up.

I next called Washington, D.C. The evacuation strategy was a miserable failure, and I was determined to call Senator David Vitter to make some recommendations. I had known the Vitter family for many years, and had once brought my family to see David when he was in the House. He might have some influence in carrying out some of my ideas.

I knew that many lives could be saved by relying on boats instead of helicopters. The authorities needed to stop preventing boaters from coming to help and, instead, recruit more to join in. The boats could cruise up and down the neighborhoods, loading up with stranded victims as they go. It was faster, more efficient, and less costly than the helicopter rescues. The other life-saving recommendation was to saturate the airwaves with information on where people could go to find dry ground or safety. The information could be sent out over the radio and from loudspeakers on boats or aircraft. Many people could save themselves if only they knew where to go. These recommendations would have been very valuable in our ordeal, shortening the evacuation by one or two days. Many of the deaths in our facility might not have occurred.

After three attempts, I finally connected to his office.

"Hi, I'm Dr. Richard Deichmann," I said. "I'm a friend of the Vitter family, and I just assisted with the evacuation of Baptist Hospital in New Orleans. I need to get in touch with David to talk with him about ways to improve the evacuation."

"Yes, sir," the staffer said. "He's very busy and communications are very bad, but we'll try to get in touch with him. How can he reach you?"

I gave him the phone number, hoping the staffer wasn't regarding me as just another crackpot constituent bitching about the conditions. I wondered if the senator would even get my message.

As it turned out, it didn't really matter. By Friday evening, the Superdome, the Convention Center, and essentially all of the inundated areas had been evacuated of most of the people who wanted to leave.

The call from David Vitter never came.

In the weeks that followed, our family tried to pick up the pieces of what remained of our lives. The most urgent decisions involved school and shelter.

Within the next twenty-four hours, we made the decision to live in Atlanta with Meredith's family. Paige and Claire could go to school there, and Meredith's house was big enough to accommodate all of us. Paige was disappointed, since many of her friends had enrolled in Grand Coteau, the local Sacred Heart school outside of Lafayette. Claire didn't care. The job prospects seemed brighter in Atlanta, too. If we liked it, we might even permanently relocate there.

So, on Sunday we loaded our meager belongings and donated clothes into the car and headed for a stop at our home in New Orleans on the way to Atlanta. Barry and Tricia came along to get things from their house too. Local police let us through a checkpoint about thirty miles outside of New Orleans and again at another checkpoint on Highway 61 outside of LaPlace, twenty miles from home. At each checkpoint, Cecile and I flashed our physician identifications. The National Guard manned the last checkpoint, about ten miles from my home. A soldier interrogated me, but let me through since I was a physician.

The long delays at the checkpoints added another two hours to the trip. Our caravan was armed with shotguns, provisioned with food and water, and stocked with two five-gallon tanks of gasoline as we entered the disaster zone. We weren't taking any chances this time.

Our home survived. A few shingles were knocked off the roof and a few windows broken in Paige's room. The flooding which had destroyed most of the region had spared our neighborhood. Two massive water oaks had tumbled to the ground, both missing our house. We cleaned out the refrigerator and made emergency repairs to the roof and windows. Cecile and the girls packed more clothes. The computers were loaded into the car along with other essentials for an exile in Atlanta. Finally, I dumped the rest of the gas in the two cars. Cecile would drive the Honda Accord; I'd bring the CRV. We hit the road again for Atlanta.

The hurricane had mangled all of the routes east, so a long detour starting out to the west was the only choice. By the time we got to Meridian, Mississippi at about nine o'clock, both of our cars were on empty. Not a single gas station had been open the entire way. We would have to wait in Meridian until gasoline arrived since we couldn't go any further if we didn't find gas soon. We desperately scouted around Meridian for gas. A Wal-Mart gas station with about sixty cars waiting in line provided our salvation. We gassed up and continued on to Atlanta that night.

Everyone we met in Atlanta was phenomenally generous to us. The girls were immediately accepted into two of Atlanta's finest schools, Marist and Holy Innocents. They chose Marist and were granted tuition waivers.

Med school friends helped me find a job in Atlanta working at Piedmont Hospital. Practicing medicine again provided a semblance of normality for me. Returning to work boosted my spirits and gave me something important and satisfying to focus my attention on.

But New Orleans always dominated our lives in one way or another. Cecile obsessed about when the girls' schools would reopen. I worried about the business state of our group, Audubon Internal Medicine, and whether we should close. Many of our friends weren't sure they would be coming back. Five physicians, including our children's pediatrician, committed suicide from the despair during those dark months. Was there enough life left in the city for us to return?

When the bodies were "discovered" at Baptist Hospital, I had been in Atlanta, steadily recovering from the trauma of the whole affair. I was surprised that there was any "discovery" at all, since I had assumed that these bodies had been retrieved shortly after my discussion with Mr. Arvin. I also puzzled over where forty-five bodies had come from. Our count had come to thirty. Maybe Dr. Skinner had not counted the bodies in Lifecare Hospital. Maybe the bodies included bodies of people who weren't patients and had been dumped there after we left.

About the same time, a doctor whom I had not met nor even seen at the hospital told CNN that he thought euthanasia might have occurred at the hospital. The Louisiana state attorney general launched an investigation to look into the allegations, which continues now more than a year after Katrina. His office called me for my story, but never did call back to actually get my statement. Reporters from around the country somehow tracked me down to get my views on the sensational story. I didn't have much to tell the media about the "euthanasia," since I didn't know anything about it.

To this day, I still wonder how forty-five bodies were found there. Did Dr. Skinner miss some of the bodies? Were bodies brought there after we left? Could it be that euthanasia really was performed? The media reports spun a sinister undertone to the valiant efforts of the men and women who worked day and night in deplorable conditions to save so many lives at the hospital. I talked with a number of the staff and physicians who had been trapped in the ordeal with me. None of us had seen or heard of anybody being euthanized at the hospital. We all wondered what was going on with the sensational euthanasia allegations. A second cycle of my feelings of abandonment and betrayal ensued.

Sentiment among Cecile, Paige, and Claire steadily shifted to a definite desire to return to New Orleans. I argued about the benefits of staying in Atlanta to an unconvinced trio. Cecile and Paige decided to go back to New Orleans as soon as Sacred Heart—her school back home—reopened in November. Claire and I stayed in Atlanta until Dominican—her high school in New Orleans—opened in January. Just before the storm, Cecile had left her job at Ochsner and accepted a position at Tulane as the director of the child psychiatry training program. She assumed her new position in a devastated program which had no patients to see, nor a facility in which to see them.

Our medical group, Audubon Internal Medicine, attempted to continue operating out of Touro Infirmary. After a very short time, we realized the financial impossibility of sustaining the business. We began negotiations with Ochsner, as well as a few other organizations in town. I drove back and forth to New Orleans so often for negotiating sessions and business meetings while working as a hospitalist in Atlanta that I felt as if I had two full-time jobs. We eventually worked out an agreement with Ochsner and moved our group to its main campus.

An independent levee investigation team found that the failure of the levees was a result of poor design and construction by the Army Corps of Engineers. The design failures were predicted by models that the Corps itself tested years before. The water broke through the porous mud levees at the Seventeenth Street Canal and the London Avenue Canal, even though the surge was four feet from the top of the levee. The water poured over the top of the Orleans Avenue Canal, where a long section was six feet lower than the rest of the levee. The commander of the Corps finally accepted responsibility for the greatest engineering failure in its history, saying that the levee protection system was one in name only.

The natural disaster of Katrina and the man-made failures of the flood that followed combined to take the lives of more than thirteen hundred people. Many bodies were washed out to sea and will never be found. New Orleanians returning home and demolition workers hauling off debris are still pulling the remains of Katrina victims from homes and attics, more than a year after the event. Hundreds, perhaps thousands, of elderly evacuees died from the evacuation itself or from the stress and strain of trying to survive in a strange new world, removed from their usual health care and familiar surroundings. At least fifteen of my elderly patients died in the three months after the storm in such circumstances. The true death toll from the largest disaster to hit this country will never be known.

A new hurricane season is upon New Orleans now. The city is moving on, though not in any particular direction. Die-hard New Orleanians have returned to rebuild in a patchwork of previously inundated neighborhoods. Crime has returned, too, at greater levels than pre-Katrina. The National Guard now patrols our streets in battle gear. Construction companies are booming. The medical infrastructure is a shell of its former self. Psychiatric services, arguably the most needed of all assistance, are practically non-existent. There's a strange demographic glut of restaurant owners but not enough dishwashers; of hotel administrators but not enough laundry workers. People chatter in Spanish working out at the health club and waiting in line at the grocery.

My demons, which had regularly haunted my nights in the months following the flood, don't come as often anymore. Tropical Storm Alberto recently swept through the Gulf of Mexico. One night, as the storm threatened, a dead man threw off the rumpled, dirty sheet covering his stiff body and arose from his stretcher. He shuffled down the Magnolia garage ramp in a ragged hospital gown to the waterline below. The bony-faced old man looked into my eyes with a pale, toothless grin and boarded a flat-bottom boat. I awoke in a cold sweat, panting. The demons are still with me, after all.

ACKNOWLEDGMENTS

The help and support of many friends and family members contributed to the conception and birth of this book. I want to first thank Meredith Many, and David and John Eatman for providing my family and me a safe harbor to dock in for the four months after the storm. Their emotional support and unselfishness in allowing us to take over their home in Atlanta make them part of that large cadre of Katrina heroes in my eyes. Steve McCollam, a timeless friend from college and med school, and Rick Fullerton, chief of the Piedmont hospitalist program, threw me a professional lifeline and set me up at their hospital. Jeff and Julie Marshall, more Atlanta friends, taught me how to laugh again during those dark days.

Many individuals at Ochsner Health System have worked to help me and my medical group re-establish ourselves professionally in New Orleans. In particular, I'd like to thank Sandy Kemmerly, Joe Dalovisio, Gloria Leary, and Richard Guthrie.

The memories could not have presented themselves as words on paper if not for the Loyola Writing Institute and Professor James Nolan, who instructed me in the art of the writing craft.

James has guided and encouraged me throughout the entire process of penning and publishing this story. Thanks as well to Maureen Jennings, who gave welcome editorial advice and criticism.

Finally, I want to thank my family for their support. Cecile and Paige made especially important suggestions and contributions. Moreover the emotional support and encouragement of my family kept me going to the end.

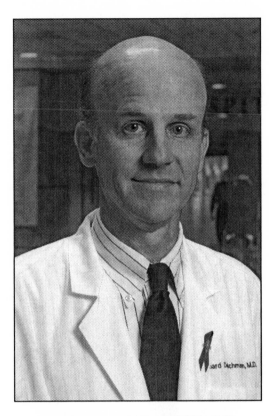

ABOUT THE AUTHOR

Richard Deichmann graduated from Tulane School of Medicine and completed his training in Internal Medicine at the University of North Carolina in Chapel Hill, North Carolina. He moved back to his hometown after completing his training in 1986, and had practiced at Baptist Hospital until Katrina. He continues his work as a physician, teacher, and clinical researcher at Ochsner Medical Center.

Dr. Deichmann, an avid triathlete, lives in the New Orleans area with his wife and three daughters.

www.rdeichmann.com

A portion of the proceeds from this book is being donated for mental health care in New Orleans.